MW00714778

Is My Child's Speech Normal?

Is My Child's Speech Normal?

. . . .

Second Edition

. . . .

JON EISENSON

pro·ed

8700 Shoal Creek Boulevard
Austin, Texas 78757-6897

pro·ed

© 1997 by PRO-ED, Inc.
8700 Shoal Creek Boulevard
Austin, Texas 78757-6897

All rights reserved. No part of the material protected by this copyright notice may be reproduced or used in any form or by any means, electronic or mechanical, including photocopying, recording, or by any information storage and retrieval system, without the prior written permission of the copyright owner.

Publisher's Note: Portions of the material in this book are adaptations of sections from *Language and Speech Disorders in Children* by J. Eisenson, 1986, Elmsford, NY: Pergamon Press. Copyright 1986 by J. Eisenson. Adapted with permission.

Library of Congress Cataloging-in-Publication Data

Eisenson, Jon, 1907–
    Is my child's speech normal? / Jon Eisenson.—2nd ed.
       p.   cm.
    Previously published : Is your child's speech normal? 1976.
    Includes bibliographical references and index.
    ISBN 0-89079-704-8 (alk. paper)
    1. Speech disorders in children.   2. Children—Language.
  I. Eisenson, Jon, 1907–   . Is your child's speech normal?
  II. Title.
RJ496.S7E38   1997
618.92′855—dc20   96-33504
                                    CIP

This book is designed in Concorde and Garamond.

Production Manager: Alan Grimes
Production Coordinator: Karen Swain
Managing Editor: Tracy Sergo
Art Director: Thomas Barkley
Reprints Buyer: Alicia Woods
Editor: Sue Motzer
Editorial Assistant: Claudette Landry
Editorial Assistant: Suzi Hunn

Printed in the United States of America

1 2 3 4 5 6 7 8 9 10   01 00 99 98 97

Contents

Prologue

When I was a child, I spake as a child, I understood as a child: But when I became a man, I put away childish things.

I CORINTHIANS, 13, 11

In the beginning there is the newly born infant, whose first sounds, which we identify as crying, are promises of more articulate sounds to come. These we may identify as "prelanguage." The crying, and later the cooing, are instinctive. For the moment let us define *instinctive* as expressing something that may send us messages, but the producer—the infant—does so without intention. Nevertheless, the various sounds—and these will increase in number—are both instinctive and species specific. The infant has joined the species Homo sapiens, also known as human beings.

Why do children "learn" to talk? There is no more reason to ask this *why* than to ask why most birds chirp or sing or make some other sound characteristic of their kind. Steven Pinker (1994), an eminent language scientist, in a rather amusing comparison of infants to spiders, answered this "nonquestion" by observing, "Spiders spin webs because they have spider brains, which give them the urge to spin and the competence to succeed" (p. 18). Pinker added, "In nature's talent show we are simply a species of primates with our own act, a knack for communicating information about who did what to whom by modulating the sounds we make when we exhale" (p. 19). I assume that Pinker means "controlled exhaled breath" to distinguish it from mere biological exhalation. There is little question that a highly developed brain with its multibillion brain cells and a unique "prewiring" gives almost all of us the capacity to understand speech and in turn to become speakers, though with varying degrees of competence.

Almost all infants who have the advantage of full-term gestation of healthy mothers and no problems in arriving on the human scene are able, according to their individual schedules, to live up to the recurrent miracle of acquiring the language of the members of their caring family. But a few, somewhat more often boys than girls, do not acquire (learn) speech by membership and exposure. Some children are so late in expressing the miracle of showing that indeed they have not been denied the "instinct" and its potentials that parents and often grandparents become anxiously concerned. This small population of children who are in fact seriously delayed in speech onset *and* understanding of spoken words are brain *different* or actually brain *damaged*. The latter are, of course, also brain different. For those who are not actually brain damaged, there may be a delay in the maturation of the "wiring system" that makes the onset of early understanding and consequent production of language possible according to anticipated schedule.

The wiring system of children who have incurred actual brain damage, by virtue of accident or disease, is not sufficiently developed—or has been disrupted in development—to allow them to learn an auditory language system by the usual exposure and interaction with caring speakers. Both of these small populations of children will be considered in this book. Happily, we can anticipate later discussions by assuring those who need to be assured that a large majority of these children are capable of learning by direct teaching.

A third group of children may come by their apparent delay in beginning to speak on an "inherited" basis. The members of this group may have relatives, often grandparents if not their own parents, who were also delayed in producing their first words, but not delayed in understanding what is said to them. These anxiety producers may respond appropriately to statements if they are interesting and not too lengthy. But the response should call for an action. For reasons not understood, they seem to be loath to put their thoughts or needs into words.

Albert Einstein is said to have been such a child. According to his biographer, Ronald Clark (1971), "The one feature of his childhood about which there appears no doubt is the lateness with which he learned to speak."

However, my own biased interpretation is that Albert as a child was waiting for some person to come along who might understand what he had to say.

It is customary in a preface or "prologue" to acknowledge and thank those who somehow, not necessarily in identified ways, contributed to this book. I will make no attempt to name individuals, but the number is legion. In that legion are the children and parents with whom I shared concerns during my professional lifetime, both in my private practice and during my tenure as director of the Queens College Speech and Hearing Center and later as director of clinics and institutes at Stanford University and San Francisco State University.

Now, for whom is this book intended? Primarily, for parents who are interested, curious, or possibly anxiously concerned that their child has not yet given expression to the recurrent miracle of spoken language. *Is Your Child's Speech Normal?* is also addressed to family physicians and pediatricians who need to know about child language so that they will have educated answers for parents who ask questions about their child's speech development. Often the question takes the following form: "Why isn't my child speaking? His sister began to speak when she was 11 months of age. Jimmy is more than twice his sister's age; what's wrong?" Perhaps the largest intended professional audience are language clinicians (speech pathologists and speech therapists) who need answers to the same questions. And last, but by no means the least in importance, are educators—nursery and kindergarten teachers as well as primary-grade teachers—who also need informed answers for themselves and parents.

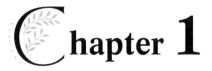

Is My Child's Speech Normal?
A Preview

"Why isn't my child talking?" "Is there a reason why my child is so slow to talk?" "I think that my child is trying to talk." "He makes sounds that sometimes resemble words, but we don't have a clue as to what he is trying to tell us." "He is almost 2 years old; why is he so late?" In my professional roles as a psychologist and speech pathologist for considerably longer than a quarter of a century, I have entertained these questions almost every working day. The questions were almost always from concerned and anxious parents. Most often the parent or parents were referred to me by a pediatrician or a previous school teacher. Almost as often, the referral came as a result of an observation by a respected friend or a relative that there is something wrong with the child's speech—that he or she should be speaking better at his or her age. Sometimes the well-intentioned adult friend or relative has merely forgotten how a child should be expected to speak at 2 or even 3 years of age, that "baby talk" is quite normal if not carried too far and too long. Often, however, the observation that the child's speech was not "right" serves to confirm the parents' own concern.

In my interview with parents, I almost always start with, "Tell me, just what is it about your child's speech that brings us together in my office?" The most frequent response is, "Johnny isn't talking right." To this, my own most likely reply is, "Try to be specific. Give me some examples of what your youngster seems to be trying to say, or what you expect him [her] to say that he [she] fails to produce."

I may then get an example or description of baby talk, or of hesitant, repetitive speech that is likely to be identified as stuttering or stammering. Less frequently, parents explain, "He seems to talk a blue streak, but it's just nonsense to us. We can't make head or tail of what he is trying to tell us. Sometimes he throws a tantrum or cries in sheer frustration. Sometimes we cry along with him."

On occasion, but much less frequently, parents inform me that their youngster was born with a damaged brain. "He's 4 years old but doesn't talk. We're not sure that he understands what we say to him." These parents want to know whether their child will ever talk well enough to be understood. "What can we do for him?"

Occasionally I am informed that their Ricky was born with a cleft palate. The palate has been repaired, but, "We still have great difficulty in understanding him. Can he be helped?"

Perhaps the most frequent complaint is, "Jorge is 2 years old, but he has only two or three words that we can understand. Mostly he grunts and points. His sister had a lot to say and said it when she was Jorge's age. What's wrong?"

All of the observations and questions raised by the parents—and my responses to them—show proper and usually justified concern. In effect, they are asking, "Is my child's speech normal?" Or, "Why isn't my child talking?" Or, "Why don't we understand what the youngster is trying to tell us?" Or, "Is there any reason to believe that our child will never be talking right?" Almost always, "What can we do to help our child talk right?" When such questions are addressed to a pediatrician, the family doctor, a child psychologist, or a specialist in language and speech, the parents have a right to replies that are not put-offs and certainly not put-downs.

In the majority of my interviews and follow-up sessions with parents, I have been able to reassure them that there was nothing significantly wrong with their child's speech that time and growing a little bit older would not correct. In some instances I recommend assistance from a speech therapist or a language clinician. Occasionally I feel the need to recommend the help of a child psychiatrist or child psychologist to get at the problem behind the immediate problem—the complaint about the child's speech. On occasion I recommend counseling for the parents (note the plural). Every so often I suggest speech or voice therapy for one or both of the parents. But before I do so, with permission, I record and play back a segment of conversation with them.

In my sessions with parents I ask many questions about the child's early health history, the child's early crying and play sounds, and the child's responses to sounds—human, animal, and mechanical. I also ask about age of walking; left-, right-, or neither-handedness; how the child keeps himself or herself occupied when awake, who talks to the child, and what happens when the child tries to talk. But the most frequent questions I ask are, "Does the child pay attention to you when you talk directly to him [or her]?" "Does the child understand you?" "How do you know?"

These are significant and key questions that will be answered in later chapters. But an early explanation is also in order.

"Normal" Varies

In a strict sense, the first of the questions, "Is my child's speech normal?" should refer only to a youngster who has begun to talk. But children tell us a great deal about their potential as listeners and speakers several months before they say their first recognizable words. They tell us about their potentials and themselves in their early crying, and in their cooing, gurgling, and babbling. The sounds they make in their early sound play are their own prologues to their future as talkers, and, not just coincidentally, as listeners, too.

We can begin to appreciate how much children understand of what we say to them by their actions—their nonverbal responses—as early as 3 months and usually no later than 6 months before they say their first words. Note that we are using a range of time and not a specific age in weeks or months. "Normal" is not a point in time but a period or range of time. *Within certain limits is normal.* Earlier than the limits is precocious. Just beyond these limits is near normal. Normal is not average, whatever that may mean. *Normal is about right.* Rarely is it exactly right in terms of a specific time.

We also need to keep in mind that no human being is at any age or at all times the same degree of "normal." Even within a range, "normal" tells us only about a child's behavior at the time we make our judgment. Some children are late starters and catch up. Often this "late start" follows a family pattern. These by far outnumber the few children who are early starters and fall behind. These relatively few children probably had something happen to them—illness, a physical or psychological traumatic event, a familial problem that demanded major adjustment—that negated the promise and prospect of an early start.

With our basic understanding that "normal" is within a range, rather than a certain age or time or a specific accomplishment, we can provide at least tentative answers to questions of parents and clinicians whom they may consult. Most of the questions center around three main points:

1. *Articulation*—How well has the child mastered the sounds of the language system?

2. *Vocabulary*—Is the youngster's vocabulary large enough to indicate needs, feelings, and thoughts?

3. *Syntax*—Is the child proficient in putting words together according to the "rules" (grammar) of the language of the home?

Authorities in language development have, over the years, made several relevant observations that provide answers to these questions. These findings, including those of the present author, are based on research with normal and as well as linguistically delayed children. These findings have important and broad implications. Following are a few of them.

• A child should begin to understand some of what is said to him or her on repeated and meaningful occasions between the ages of 6 and 9 months. Exceptions are children who are deaf, severely hard of hearing, or mentally slow. A child may show understanding by behavior as simple as a change of position, such as getting ready to be picked up, or when mother or daddy says, "Up baby," or, "Now baby, up," or, "Up we go," and so on. The child should, unless disinclined to respond, change posture when the words alone are spoken, even before or along with the picking-up gesture. Similarly, the child may offer a hand on the request, "Give me your hand, darling," or look expectantly for father if mother says, "Here comes daddy."[1] Most children who are going to talk—perhaps up to 90%—begin their careers as talkers (say their first words) by 15 months of age. Some produce their first words as early as 9 months, and a few precocious ones, more likely to be girls than boys, as early as 8 months.

---

[1]Children who are deaf and whose parents use sign language learn comparable signs within the same range of time as hearing children respond to words.

• The first words need not be of adult form. Any sound combination that is produced fairly regularly to label or identify a person, thing, or event is acceptable as a first word. Thus, *wawa* will do for *water*, *doddy* or *goggy* for *doggy*, and *buh-buh* or *doh-doh* for *daddy*. (Note the repetition of sounds. This is a feature of early language.) Mothers, happily, are more likely to be "mama," or some production close to it, than are fathers to be called "dada." When a child begins to talk, it is she or he who determines the form of the word that the adult must gracefully accept. However, this acceptance does not impose a need for the adult to use the same early language forms as the child.

• In a few weeks, perhaps a month or two, after the child has begun to build up a vocabulary for labeling or naming, she or he is likely to use some of the same words, and a few new ones, to make things happen. These "command" words are used as tools to bring things about, to meet developing needs. The same words are still used as labels for what is present or to identify what is happening that is of interest to him or to her. Words are now the forerunners of events, while they continue to be the names of objects, actions, or persons the child wants. Thus, the child calls (announces) "mommy"—or the equivalent in his or own articulation—when mother is wanted, even when she may be out of sight; or "wawa" to get some fluid, or demand "doddy" to get his or her doll or stuffed animal, or even shout "up" to be picked up or taken out of the crib or playpen. The voice of command has a different intonation than the voice for naming. This difference the child learns from listening to the grown-ups to whom he or she relates.

• About the time that a child has vocabulary of from 50 to 60 words used as labels or as demands, she or he usually begins to combine some of them into two-word "statements." For a majority of children, this occurs by 18 months (obviously, at a later time if the child is a late starter in beginning to talk). Typical infant sentences take the form of "baby up" or "baby wawa" or "baby mommy." Each statement indicates what the child wants as well as expects to happen, or else what it is an announcement for!

• The child's comprehension of language, from the very beginning, exceeds his or her ability to speak. This continues to be so for all of us throughout the life span. This is so for both day-to-day discourse and writing.

These guideposts, intended primarily for parents directly or by way of a professional whom the parents may consult, should not only help to inform but also help, in most instances, to relieve anxiety about the question, "Is my child's speech normal?" Later we will expand on these guidelines and raise and answer other questions and issues about degrees of normality—about children who seem to be "laws unto themselves," who are slow to speak but who catch up as they grow from infancy to childhood. We will also consider other children for whom concern is very much in order, and what actions to take to reduce what may otherwise become serious delay in talking, thinking, and learning.

Each Child Is an Individual

Each of us has an individual way of speaking—including young children. By the time a child is 4 years of age, he or she speaks the language of the grown-ups close to her or him, but still manages to speak in a distinctive way that is somehow different from all other speakers of the same language. Each child learns words, mostly the words of older speakers with whom she or he has meaningful contact. Nevertheless, each child has favorite words or phrases, and favorite ways of turning a phrase or sentence in making statements and asking questions. Each child has an "idiolect."

Although a normal human being reflects the influence of others in learning a language, no human being is a clone or replica of any other person, regardless of how important the other person may be in his or her life.

Human beings are members of a species that, if normal, are endowed with the capacity to learn to talk. Psychologists, anthropologists, and other persons who qualify as authorities on the matter of learning to talk sum up their observations on learning to talk in a variety of ways and often in technical terms that identify their professions. But, in simplest form, their observations come down to, "Human beings acquire speech because that is what it means, at a minimum, to be human." Of course, we know that *some* human beings *do not* talk. And a few elect, at least from time to time, not to talk. We also know that those who do learn to talk vary considerably in this distinctively and uniquely human achievement.

Why some children are unable to learn to speak by exposure to speakers —to learn without being aware early in life that they are learning—will be considered later. There are causes and reasons for a child's late onset of talking, for slowness in understanding spoken language, for defective speech, and for absence of speech, as well as speech that defies ready comprehension even by well-intentioned listeners.

Beginning with the birth cry, there are numerous signs that reveal and project whether and when in childhood a child may begin to understand spoken language and become a speaker. There are also indicators, fortunately not carved in stone, that may indicate how capable, or at least how close to "normal," he or she will be in beginning to talk. This is not to claim that we can make predictions with anything close to certainty; we would be wise to leave a margin for error in projecting estimates.

We now know considerably more about how children acquire language, and what they acquire as they mature as speakers, than we did even as recently as the 1970s. Accordingly, a professional person responsible for providing guidance to parents about their children is obligated to know whereof he or she speaks when "advising" parents with, "Don't worry, everything will be all right. I have known children who did not begin to talk until age 3 years."

To be sure, some children are early talkers and others are late talkers. But mere chance is not the determining factor. There are fewer late understanders of speech than there are late talkers. Some children follow a family pattern of not talking until the age of 3 years and a few, very few, to 3^1/$_2$ years of age. But no child with normal hearing is late in listening to understand what a parent or other caretaker is saying directly to that child with well-chosen words rather than a flow of utterances that overwhelms the would-be listener.

The child who is an early talker is not likely to be a cause of concern to parents. But the exceptionally late talker may, quite legitimately, be a cause for concern—not only to the parents but also to the professional advisor.

Help for Children with Problems

In later chapters, we shall consider in some detail the recurrent miracle of the development of spoken language. We shall talk about what parents can do to enhance their child's speech acquisition, as well as what they should avoid doing: When "lay off" is the best policy and when "it's time to get going." We shall consider problems such as cluttered speech and stuttering, deviant articulation, inappropriate or defective voice production, and the special problems of children who have severe hearing loss as well as those with impaired physical mechanisms for the production of speech. We shall also consider the child, and the parents of the child, who has difficulty in relating to other human beings and either does not talk or whose use of language does not communicate a comprehensible message.

We shall be informed to whom to turn when advice and help are needed. In this regard, we shall learn how to distinguish between the competent professional person and the well-intentioned and usually unqualified nonprofessional, or the person operating out of his or her professional field. In sum, this book not only answers the question, "Is my child's speech normal?" but it also provides information about what to do, where to go, and whom to consult, if for some reason the answer to the question is not a clear and confident "yes."

Considerably more can be done today for children who are slow or deviant speakers than could be done for their parents or grandparents when they were children. Our present knowledge enables us to identify potential problems in language development and speech production at an early age. Three related professional disciplines are available to us to deal with children and their parents who need help.

Speech and language clinicians are specialists in the diagnosis of speech and language problems. Usually they work on a one-to-one basis with their clients. Some may offer services to small groups whose members have the same problems. In some areas of the United States, the term *speech pathologist,* or *speech correctionist* is used as a synonym for *speech and language clinician.* Whatever the term used—in England and Europe they have different names—these professionals treat young children who are developmentally deficient in acquiring spoken language and becoming proficient speakers. They also help those who, as a result of injury or disease, have suffered damage to their initially normal capacity to comprehend and produce speech.

Audiologists are specialists in hearing, both normal and deficient. Audiologists are concerned with assessing hearing capacity for spoken language, the identification of hearing loss, as well as treatment of persons with impaired hearing. *Teachers of the deaf* are educators who work with children who are deaf, usually in school settings. Preschool children may be treated individually or in small groups.

These professionals—speech and language clinicians (speech pathologists), audiologists, and teachers of the deaf—have learned a great deal since their specialties first developed in the 1920s and 1930s. Although learning is ongoing, they are aware of what they do not know as well as what they are confident they know. Moreover, the persons in these related fields are usually members of professional organizations that recommend or require standards of education and training that include supervised training for certification and employment. All of these professions publish journals to disseminate information based on research and individual experience. A majority of the states have established licensing requirements for their professional practitioners and teachers. Because of these requirements, children and their parents are now better served than ever before.

In the next few chapters, we will follow the child from the first cry and pleasure sounds to first words and then to sentences. In these chapters I will address myself to the primary question, "Is my child's speech normal?" Later chapters will consider children less likely to be within the range we consider normal, as well as children who are seriously deficient in the comprehension and therefore, inevitably, in the production of spoken language.

If you are a parent, I hope that you will find much in this book that will help you to have positive feelings about the future of your child as a listener and speaker, even if your youngster admittedly has problems. Few—very few—problems are beyond help if identification and treatment are initiated at the right time with the right professional persons. If you are one of the professional persons, I hope that the information in this volume will serve as a guide in your consultation with concerned parents.

$\mathcal{C}$hapter 2

From the First Cry to the First Word

Infant Crying

When in pain or discomfort, all creatures who are capable of making a noise do so. Children are no exception. They differ from all other noise-making creatures in variety of noises, including crying, that they learn to produce. Children, and of course adolescents and adults, also learn to make noises—sounds and later words—that express their state of comfort or of satisfaction and pleasure. But for the time being, we will stay with infants and share observations on the sounds we identify as crying.

The way children cry[1] tells us whether all is going well, or whether conditions need correcting. One condition for the newborn infant and for the first month of life may be that he or she is not breathing properly or needs some help to get going. Soon other cries inform the mother or other caretaker that an empty tummy is not a happy tummy, or that baby needs a debubbling, a change of linen, or merely a change of position in the crib. Rarely does an infant engage in crying without reason.

We affirm this despite what parents, relatives, and especially close-by neighbors may assert to the contrary. Unfortunately, infants cannot explain

---

[1]We will use the word *cry* to include comfort sounds as well as the sounds they make when crying.

their crying. By the time the child is old enough to provide explanations, he or she does not need to resort to crying. But some do, perhaps just to keep in practice. If crying persists, the child may be showing us that she or he has somehow learned that crying is more effective than talking in getting one's way, in getting attention, or in getting rid of what is not wanted.

How should babies cry? Lustily and loud enough to show that they mean it. This kind of crying informs us that physiologically, at least, all is well.[2] The doctor who delivers the baby may have to give the newborn a sharp whack on the backside to get him or her to breathe and, as a consequence, announce it by crying. This is reflexive crying. No matter what cynical philosophers may wish to believe, the newborn infant does not intend to cry. Babies may and do cry because they cannot help themselves. For the moment, it is painful to have to breathe on one's own. It hurts because mother-warmed vocal cords have become a bit chilled now that the baby no longer has the protection of the mother's body. The infant cries because the change in climate in the new external environment causes the vocal cords to contract suddenly. As the newborn does his or her first solo breathing, the vocal cords are set into motion. This, too, hurts a bit, and so the infant cries. The baby is responding reflexively to all of the sudden changes in her or his conditions of life.

How should babies cry? Normal babies cry much alike, but still not exactly alike. A characteristic cry—a good cry—usually has three identifiable phases. In the first phase, the infant seems to be tentative about crying and appears to be trying out the vocal apparatus, as well as his or her intentions, by a barely audible whimper or two. The infant is tuning up, preparing for the next phase.

In the second phase, the baby goes all out, possibly because she or he has been frightened with the intensity of the vocal behavior. What begins as a just-audible "wa-wa," "naa-naa," "ai-ai," or a variety of such repeated sounds increases to a sustained loud crescendo that may change from a low-pitched to a high-pitched tone. After this, the infant may pause for just a moment and then start anew. This vocal performance may be repeated again, and yet again.

---

[2]Some babies are colicky. In his book *Crybabies,* Weissbluth (1984, p. 13) defined colic as "inconsolable crying for which no physical cause can be found, which lasts more than 3 hours a day, occurs at least 3 days a week and continues for at least 3 weeks."

In the third phase, the baby sounds as if she or he is petering out, at least for the time being. The baby may well be finished with crying if the parent or other familiar caregiver corrects whatever may have caused the crying in the first place. If nothing effective is done, perhaps because the mother or other caregiver did not correctly guess what was needed to comfort the child, the crying will be resumed. The third phase may well be a warning that means, "I'm putting you on alert. Guess again. Now you must do whatever is necessary to make me comfortable. If you don't, there's more where this came from."

If the baby cries in these three stages and gives you the message, "I'm about to cry, I'm crying, I'm about to stop but I can go at it again," be grateful. He or she is making a good start toward becoming a normal talker. The baby's first crying sounds, like most first activities, are spasmodic and not under control. They are reflexive and, in a very real sense, they control the child. If you have the courage, watch what is taking place when a baby cries. You will probably note that when the baby is crying beyond the first phase, it is a total body affair. The entire body is at work, legs and arms in motion, facial muscles contracted. Literally, the infant is crying all over.

What about the baby who cries with a mere whimper and then stops? What of the "good baby" who rarely ever cries and seems content to be alone, even when awake? We shall consider these babies later. At the present time we will only suggest that babies *should* cry, that normal babies *do* cry, and that almost all of them do so in the manner we have described. If the baby cries too little, or too much, or merely whimpers in a token manner, consult the child's doctor. Parents have a right to be assured that all is well, or to be informed of what they should do if all is not well.

Assuming that the baby is born full term and that everything goes smoothly, we can anticipate changes in crying after the first 3 or 4 weeks. During the first few weeks the baby cries with a limited repertoire of sounds. He or she is usually a virtuoso only in regard to loudness. When hungry, the infant may combine loud volume and pitch in a rhythmic production that accompanies the contractions and relaxations of an empty tummy. All we can guess from the baby's vocal performance other than the hunger cry is that he or she is uncomfortable or in actual pain. But the crying all sounds alike, so that not even a loving mother or a doting grandmother can do anything but guess at the cause of the discomfort. A need for a change of linen is a likely exception, because it may stimulate senses other than hearing in the observer.

The Sounds Before the Words

Crying and Cooing in Many Keys

Beginning with the second month, the baby can express considerably more via crying than he or she did as a newborn. Part of the baby's waking time is spent in making sounds that, as fond parents, we refer to as *cooing*. Though some of the sounds do resemble the cooing of the dove, most are more varied and more interesting. In an important way, the sounds of the cooing stage seem to be under the baby's control. In the first 4 weeks the occasional grunting and gurgling noises sound like by-products of digestive activity. (Perhaps that is why Shakespeare referred to the infant as "mewling and puking in the nurse's arms.") But beginning in the second month, if the baby has had the benefit of a full-term pregnancy and a normal delivery, he or she makes sounds to signal that all is well in the world. The infant also makes considerably more vehement and strident sounds to signal that all is not well. Some of these discomfort sounds are now sufficiently different from one another that they convey what is wrong. Now the hunger cry is different from the gas-in-the-tummy cry and from the cry that ceases when the baby is turned over, or has his or her linen changed, or has the bed coverings rearranged to give room for arms and legs to move.

In a very important way, both the crying and the cooing tell parents something about their baby's state of being. Though the baby's sound making is still reflexive, without conscious intent, the child is nevertheless sending informative signals. These signals, because they are different from one another, reduce the amount of guessing that the baby's parents need to do. We now have the important beginnings of communication.

One of the things the baby's crying and cooing tell us (whether or not we are parents) is how the baby is feeling about himself or herself while vocalizing. This component of the message will continue throughout life. By our tone of voice, by the way we sound, we reveal how we truly feel about what we say. Just as our words tell what we are thinking, our voice tells how we feel about the thoughts we are sharing. It takes the skill of an accomplished actor or a thoroughly practiced liar to make the voice conceal rather than reveal our feelings. The infant's vocalizations are sincere—his or her voice reflects and reveals current feelings to the sympathetic listener.

Cooing: The Comfort Sounds

What do the comfort sounds, the so-called cooings, tell us? Can we really describe these sounds? It is easier to answer the first question than the second. For one thing, comfort sounds tell us that the infant is a sound maker who is capable of revealing that "I'm OK" as well as "I need help to become OK." The comfort sounds also tell us that the child is maturing, that the child has the neurological and physical equipment to reveal his or her general state of being. The baby is capable, even though not yet aware of it, of communicating broad-based messages to those who will listen. And if those who listen respond, the capability will be encouraged and nurtured, and the child will mature.

How can we describe the sounds of the child who is cooing in comfort? Charles Van Riper, a colleague and authority on speech, wrote:

> The sounds used in these early comfort-vocalizations are often indescribable. You cannot spell them in any alphabet save that of love. Perhaps some of those which baffle our attempts to transcribe them are sounds used by strange or primitive tribes. After all, the baby doesn't know what language he is going to have to use. For all he knows, it may be Hottentot. We have heard good Swedish umlaut, vowels and pure Gaelic consonants in their utterance. (Van Riper, 1950, p. 15)

All babies, regardless of the culture into which they are born, or the language or languages spoken in their particular culture, cry and coo much alike.

The name that parents give to the noncrying sounds that the baby makes depends, perhaps, as much on their attitude as on the actual sounds the baby makes. So, depending partly on point of view, the baby may be said to grunt or gurgle, hiccough or cluck, babble or bubble, coo, snort, or squeal. Nevertheless, there are differences that objective nonrelatives of a particular baby can discern. In truth, the baby can and does grunt, gurgle, hiccough, cluck, babble, bubble, coo, snort, squeal, and breathe heavily with accompanying vocalization.

What the infant does is a result of how he or she feels, a reflexive by-product of the baby's physiological state. *How much* the infant does may well be a result of your attention and your responses. The more you respond, the longer the nonverbal "dialogue" will continue. Thus the parent does have some influence on the amount of the baby's sound making, if not on the specific sounds.

Those of us who speak British or American English are likely to identify several English vowels and a few English consonants in a baby's crying or cooing vocabulary. The vowels most frequently identified (many others are heard but not identified or remembered) include the long $\bar{e}$ as in *knee*, *i* as in *it*, *e* as in *wet*, and the *a* of *hat*. All these sounds are produced with the front of the tongue arched and active. Phoneticians (experts in the sound patterns of a language) call them *front vowels*. Interestingly, the baby is not likely to produce the long $\overline{oo}$ as in *coo* until he or she is 3 or 4 months of age.

Another note of interest is that the vowel sounds produced in a state of comfort have little or no nasal quality. This is so even for children of French-speaking parents, who speak "through the nose" much more than normal speakers of English. In English-speaking cultures, we associate talking through the nose with whining, with unpleasant states. As Van Riper (1950) has observed: "Unpleasantness usually uses the trombone of the nose for its expression, but contentment comes out of the mouth" (pp. 15–16). Playing these different tunes on a conscious and controlled level is something that the child must learn to do. But from 1 month of age to 3 or 4 months, the tunes come naturally, spontaneously, and sincerely.

Babbling

Two or three months after the child has become a part-time awake but not-crying sound maker, he or she is likely to begin true *babbling*. Now the child, usually by 16 to 20 weeks of age, seems to be listening to the sounds produced, and may repeat a few of these productions. If we view this behavior generously, we may note that the child occasionally smiles or makes an approving gurgling noise after one of these renditions.[3] Sometimes such divinely inspired oral renditions take place just before the baby falls asleep, and so the parents are likely to miss them. They are worth a secret tape recording.

Sometime between 4 to 8 months, most children begin to babble in earnest. Though some nonobjective listeners hear sounds that resemble words, the patterns of sounds are indeed languagelike but are still unintentional.

---

[3] There is little doubt that parents who speak non-European languages are more attuned to the sounds of their own speech than to the sounds of other languages. In listening, we perceive what we are inclined to hear unless we are trained to be aware of the sounds of other languages.

Babbling is intuitive sound making—evidence, if you will, for the assumption that there is a language instinct. Another way of stating this point is that language is human species specific, and the child has come aboard. For the time being, we will assume that the sounds of babbling have no other identified significance.

What are the most likely sounds of babbling? Initially, as we noted, infants are internationalists and have a wide-ranging repertoire of speechlike sounds. Increasingly, however, the repertoire is narrowed to include more of the speech sounds of speakers with whom they have most contact. The most likely sounds are single stop consonants (sounds that stop the flow of breath, e.g., *p, b, t, d, k,* and *g*). These sounds may be combined with vowels, which gives us *ma, pa, da,* and *ga.* At about 6 months, most children may duplicate sounds and produce *mama, pappa,* and *gaga.*

If babbling has no intended meaning, then why do infants babble? Naomi Baron (1992, p. 51) provided an explanation if not a reason: "Largely for the same reason they crawl and turn over and throw things out of the crib: to exercise bodies and explore the world. Listen to—and watch a 6- or 7-month-old—babbling. His mouth has the plasticity of an accordion: opening and closing, narrowing and widening. . . . and then the articulators go to work."

Babbling in the early stages is very much a private (solo) affair. Babbling, or any other form of sound making, for that matter, is likely to be interrupted by the intrusion of another sound maker. Unfortunately, babbling is likely to stop altogether if interrupted, while crying is only momentarily impeded.

But after the child has practiced babbling for a month or two, the presence of another babbler may result in a social dialogue rather than silence or crying. The second participant, however, must be careful not to overwhelm the baby with a flood of oral noises. Gently and easily is the way if babbling is to be encouraged. Incidentally, each babbler says his or her own thing. Each encourages the other, but the sounds and the "music" are unrelated.

After the child has begun to babble—to produce repetitive or nearly repetitive sounds and syllables—he or she may still resort to cooing. Babies do not entirely give up the behavior of an earlier stage when they advance to a new one. They can always "regress" to an earlier stage, according to their needs. Normally babbling, as a new and identifiable stage, and later self-repetitive imitation (lalling), lasts until 6 to 8 months of age.

Lalling is speech sound repetition. Babbling tells us that the child has the necessary equipment to make speech sounds and that making a variety of sounds is fun. Lalling—the repetition of sounds that initiate with the child, such as "la-la-la," "da-da-da," or "na-na-na"—tells us not only that the child enjoys sound making but also that he or she hears the sounds and can control their production by repetition. The child is in control of his or her sound making and finds this achievement good. This is self-reinforcement!

Many parents are concerned about whether their baby really is hearing vocal sounds and other noises in a normal way. This is especially so if there are other children or relatives with hearing problems. Perhaps their baby is unusually quiet or unresponsive when spoken to. How can concerned and anxious parents determine whether there is a real hearing problem? Or a problem in attending? And if there seems to be a problem, what can they do about it? The following information should help.

Children who are deaf, or hard-of-hearing (for no child is completely without hearing), begin to babble at about the same age and under the same conditions as children who hear normally. Moreover, they sound much the same as normal babies. By the end of the fifth or sixth month, however, the deaf baby makes fewer sounds than the hearing child. Both the quantity and the variety of babbling are considerably less in deaf babies than in normal ones. Further, the deaf child's babblings are self-started. He or she does not engage in dialogue, nor does the deaf infant respond to another babbler.

Presumably, children who are deaf are quieter because they lack the normal and adequate feedback that comes from hearing their own speech and that of others. The feedback obtained by feeling the movements of the tongue and lips is ordinarily not enough to keep babbling going or to initiate lalling. In the absence of the ability to hear as well as feel the sounds they produce, these children tend to become silent unless they are made to feel uncomfortable. Even then, the sounds they produce are likely to be those made in the early babbling period, with a flat and nasal quality.

But babbling is very important, even for those who are hard-of-hearing. Eventually the child will learn to speak, and his or her speaking apparatus needs to be kept in "good running order." Babbling needs to be encouraged. This is a special problem with children suspected of having a severe hearing loss. They should be referred to a clinician who has the authority born of knowledge and experience with young children (see Chapter 13).

In addition, parents can encourage their baby's babbling by arranging a mirror or mirrors above the crib. Then the baby can not only feel but also see himself or herself talking, and the babbling stage is not only encouraged but sustained and possibly prolonged. The infant keeps the apparatus for sound making in good shape. To the limits of his or her hearing, the baby is also practicing listening.

Of course, the babbling–lalling stage is extremely important to all speech development, from its beginning as a "private affair" on through its development into social dialogue. You can encourage this normal sequence by gentle participation. Do not overwhelm the baby by a torrential flow of oral noises. Babbling, and later, lalling, indicates that the child has a working feedback system and that all is probably going well with speech development.

Sound Imitation: The Echoic Stage

Beginning at about 8 months—the range may be from 7 to 9 or even 10 months —most children begin to imitate some of the sounds and even short words they hear other people making. Lalling and babbling, both self-initiated, are of course likely to continue. In the echoic stage, the child *sounds as if he or she is talking.* If mother says "mama" or "baby," the child responds with either a remarkable imitation or one very close to what was said. At this stage, the baby has a real capacity for echoing what he or she hears, or at least part of it. However, though the child may utter "ma-ma," "da-da," or even "bye-bye," the child probably doesn't mean what he or she seems to be saying. The child does not indicate that *mama* is intended by looking at her, nor does the child look in the direction through which mama is likely to enter the room. If the baby's actions were appropriate for the echoic words, the child would then be speaking. He or she would be using verbal labels for one or two somebodies, or one or two things. But that is the next stage of speech development.

Although the child is not yet speaking—truly speaking—he or she is learning to listen to and understand the language spoken in the immediate environment. He or she responds to some names and even to some directions when others speak, and will turn to mother and to daddy, or to a doll or teddy bear, on hearing the appropriate name. The child will get ready to be picked up, provided, of course, that he or she is in the mood, when mother or daddy or another trusted adult says, "Up," or, "Up baby." The child may hug a favorite doll when that is suggested, or may reach out when asked, "Do you want your doll?" Probably the child is responding to a key word of the statement or question, but at the same time is responding and building up a comprehension vocabulary. The child is involved in the game of language!

First Words

When children produce their first true words—words that have intention and meaning—they begin in earnest to make it clear that spoken language is human species specific. They now share their thinking in words. In their choice of words, and in the manner of presenting them, they are also expressing themselves in a personalized way, in what I refer to as an *individuolect*. In their language acquisition, they progress from the single word "up" to "baby up," to "doddy (dolly) up," to a stated observation such as, "Jones knew everything he was taught, but unfortunately, that is all he ever knew." The last, of course, is an adult leap.

Now, with admiration and respect, let us review the identifiable milestones in language acquisition.

Children who speak normally usually begin to show understanding of spoken language addressed directly to them by 9 months of age. This language is usually a polite "command" or direction such as, "Open your mouth," or, "Give me your hand." By 2 years of age, the great majority of children who will be normal speakers have begun their speaking careers. Some begin by about 9 months; most begin by 15 months. Notice—and this is a very important point—that there are two parts to the language game, *understanding* and *speaking*. The child who says only a few words but understands many words should be no cause for concern, even at age 2½ years.

If the child understands what is said, there is less cause for concern than if the child neither understands nor talks. But even if the child understands speech, there is reason for *concern* and *action* if the child is not talking by age 3 years.[4]

Why some children are early starters and others are late starters is not yet clear. There is a tendency for the age of onset of talking to run in fami-

---

[4]We know a boy who did not begin to speak until he was 3½ years of age. This, of course, is exceptional. However, there was no question that he understood what his parents said to him. He indicated this by following directions and doing "errands" in his home. He was adept with tools, cut with scissors, and assembled a jigsaw puzzle as quickly as his father. But he did not seem to need to share his thoughts. He graduated from high school and entered college at age 14 years. At age 21 he earned a medical degree. At 25 he completed his residency in psychiatry. No telling how a late talker may turn out!

lies. When the tendencies run the same on both sides of the family, we are likely to have less anxiety than when mother's side has early talkers and daddy's side is somewhat slower. Later, especially in Chapter 4, we shall go into factors that are related to the onset of talking.

The late-speaking child who is from a family of early speakers (especially if he or she is late to understand speech) needs to be considered differently from the late-speaking or even nonspeaking child from a family of late speakers. However, all children who are not deaf should understand speech by 15 months. Those who do not are special children who need and deserve special consideration. But we are getting a bit ahead of ourselves. We still have an important last stage for the child to go through before he or she becomes a full-fledged multiple-word producer. We should be mindful that even though the child may be saying a few single words, labeling people, things, and perhaps a few events, he or she is likely to continue echoic speech. Frequently, if only for the fun of it, the child will indulge in babbling and lalling.

By 18 months our typical child, no longer an infant or even a baby, really arrives at the magic of language. Now the child utters the commands "mama," "dada," "milk," or "doddy" in order to get what he or she wants. The child is not naming, but is giving orders! And as these orders are obeyed, the child begins to appreciate how powerful and how potent he or she can be as a speaker. We refer to this stage as *anticipatory language,* in which the child tries to influence future events. It is true speech.

Anticipatory language is indeed true speech! There are some children, mostly among those with severe mental retardation, who may reach the *labeling* or *naming* stage but fail to progress beyond it. But when the child uses language to bring about an event, he or she changes the situation, rather than just naming or identifying it. The child also reveals that some thinking has gone on. We may assume that on the basis of a rudimentary inner language system, by talking to himself or herself, the child has rehearsed possible things to say. After the rehearsal, the child decides to speak and await results. If the results are what the child expected, the specific effort and the mode of behavior are both reinforced. If calling "mama" brings mother, and if she is what the child wanted and still wants, then speaking is worth doing. If announcing "doddy" brings dolly or doggy more quickly than "I'll grunt and you guess," then the child has a pay-off for this new ability. So, of course, has the related adult.

Many children reveal highly individual styles in their early pronouncements. The styles are incorporated into their individuolects as their inventory of spoken words increases. Our son, shortly after he was aware that he could stand on his hind legs, literally bellowed his commands. When he announced "Ball," his voice and his manner indicated that "Ball" was not to be regarded as a polite request. "Ball" meant either "I don't see my ball" or "I see my ball, but I can't get it." It also implied, "You get it and give it to me." This, we recognize, is a considerable amount to say with a single word. When his mother gave him the ball, again he announced, from the kingdom of his playpen and standing upright, "Ball." This time his pronouncement meant, "Let's play a game. You give me the ball and I'll throw it away." This, you may recognize, is a variation of the game we play with a trained dog. But the rule of turn taking is reversed. We might speculate on who is training whom.

Our daughter revealed another style. She seemed very ladylike in asking for "doddy." When her mother gave her the dolly, she smiled approvingly, looked down at her companion, again said "doddy," turned on her side, and closed her eyes for her nap. Within a week she said, "Doddy seep." This may have meant, "Give me my dolly and we'll both take a nap," or "Give me my dolly, it's time for my nap. You're dismissed." We never found out which of the two meanings was correct. By the time our daughter was old enough and had language enough to tell us, she had forgotten.

So it is with much of what the child intends by early pronouncements. We can only guess at meanings according to the circumstances. If the child behaves as if satisfied, we can assume that the meaning we guessed at was correct. At least, it was acceptable and satisfactory to the child. By our own behavior, by our guesses, we reinforce the meaning or meanings our children develop for the words they produce. And as we have observed, a single word may have multiple meanings.

With this magical power comes a new responsibility. Once a child shows us that he or she can speak, we expect the child to speak. Sometimes this is more than the child bargained for, but he or she learns soon enough that only within limits can one have one's own way. The guessing game holds only for what the child has not yet put into words. But once a child expresses wishes and feelings, he or she is held responsible for more of the same. It is up to the parents to make "more of the same" worthwhile. If not, the child may regress to earlier stages when, though things may not have been promptly obtained, life may have been a bit easier and perhaps even a bit better.

All the early stages in speech development, from early crying to the imperious stage of anticipatory speech, are summarized in Table 2.1. It also shows what physical skills the baby can be expected to have at each stage of speech development.

Table 2.1

Milestones from Birth to 18 Months

Approximate Age	Baby Says	Baby Responds
Birth– 4 weeks	Cries whenever uncomfortable, with no apparent difference in crying because of the specific cause.	Cries, eats, or sleeps. Most physical (motor) behavior involves the entire body. Flailing movements of arms and legs when crying.
4–16 weeks	Coos and makes "laughing" noises. Vocal play produces vowels and some consonant sounds involving tongue and lip activity. May engage in vocal "dialogue" with mother.	Shows awareness and need for human sounds, turns head in the direction of the source of the sound. Usually is able to support head when lying "face down." By end of this period, is likely to discover and inspect own hand.
20–24 weeks	Vocalizes when comfortable. Vowel-like cooing and considerable babbling, with consonants modifying the identifiable vowels. Makes some nasal sounds (*m, n*) and some lip sounds, including lip vibrations suggesting a "Bronx cheer."	Sits up with support. Arm and leg movements better controlled. May be able to pick up a cube.
6–7 months	Babbling now includes self-imitation (lalling). Many of the sound productions resemble one-syllable utterances that may include *ma, da, di,* and *do.*	Sits without props, using hands if necessary for support. Increased skill in picking up objects. Can reach with either hand. Smiles at own image.
8–9 months	Considerable self-imitative sound play. Is also likely to imitate (*echo*) syllables, words, and intonation patterns of older speakers.	Can stand up, holding onto an object for support. Can grasp a small object with thumb in apposition. Can pull a string to get an object.

(Continues)

Table 2.1 Continued.

Approximate Age	Baby Says	Baby Responds
10–11 months	Repeats the words of others with increased proficiency. Responds appropriately to many word cues for familiar things and "happenings." The precocious child may have several words in his (more likely *her*) vocabulary.	Indicates understanding of many verbal directions by appropriate behavior. Cooperates in games. Can pull self up to a standing position. May take side step while holding onto fixed object.
12 months	Still likely to imitate the speech of others, but so proficiently that he or she sounds as if he or she has quite a lot to say. First labeling (identification) words for most children.	May stand without support. May walk if held by one hand. Some children may take first steps alone. Most will "walk" on hands and feet.
By 18 months	Increases word inventory, possibly from 3 to 50 words. Vocalizations reveal intonational (melody) pattern of adult speakers. May begin to use two-word utterances.	Walks without support. Runs. Can manage cubes well enough to build a two-block tower. May begin to show hand preference. Can throw a ball and turn pages of a book.

Note. Note that the milestone ages are *approximate*. As a general guide, for functions related to development and age, it is wise to consider ±2 (months) for projected accomplishments. For children known to be premature, the age of expectation should be further extended by at least a month for each month of maturity. In regard to language, by age 9 months, unless there is evidence of brain damage or brain difference, the matter of prematurity should be minimal. Adapted from *Language and Speech Disorders in Children* (pp. 23–24) by J. Eisenson, 1989, New York, Pergamon Press.

Helping the Child Get Off to a Good Start

It is the rare and truly exceptional child who needs to be *taught* to talk. Almost all children acquire language the same way that song birds "learn" to sing, or so-called talking birds "learn" to imitate human speakers. The method is simply to expose the child to a speaker or speakers with whom he or she can identify. Then the child will unconsciously imitate the speech heard. The imitation is, of course, not complete. The child selects from all sounds heard only those that he or she can produce. The result is infant speech. Later, in ways that are still mysterious, the magic of infant speech gives way to the supermagic of adult speech. Sounds become sharpened and words more readily identifiable. The child also learns the way we string words together to make statements and ask questions. This last process we call "grammar," or syntax.

What kind of environment encourages a child to speak? Most simply stated, it is one in which there is talking, but not a Tower of Babel. The talking should suggest pleasure or comfort, rather than anger or discomfort. When you are talking directly to a baby, use short and simple statements. Punctuate the flow of talk with short pauses. The pauses should be frequent and well spaced, so that the child is not overwhelmed by the quantity of sounds to which he or she is directly exposed.

The child's parents and the other people who care for the child should speak as they feed, burp, change the child's linen, or whatever. They should describe what they are doing in single words or short phrases. Thus "dolly," "milk," or "cookie" may be starters. Phrases such as "baby's doll," "milk-baby," or "baby-cookie" may follow. If you have an urge to make a complete statement, "Here's your dolly" or "Up we go" are fine. But avoid long and involved observations, such as "Baby wants her dolly now, doesn't she?" Such a half statement, half question is too complicated for a young child to manage.

If you follow these suggestions—and for most parents, this approach is easy and natural—then there is little else you need to be concerned about. However, because some parents may still be concerned, here are a few additional observations.

• We want to emphasize that, in acquiring language, each child develops at his or her own rate. A slower than "average" rate of language acquisition does not mean that the child is retarded. (The exceptions, as indicated earlier, are only for children who do not comprehend speech, children who cannot hear, or children who in other ways indicate that they are severely mentally retarded.)

• Some children add to their comprehension and speaking vocabularies in increments that are almost regular and predictable. Other children progress by spurts and tantalizing plateaus. Most plateaus, however, are periods when the child is consolidating previous gains. A great deal is going on inside that is not readily apparent in the child's outward speech and behavior.

• In deciding how well their child's speech is developing, parents would be wise to assume 1 month's leeway up to a year of age, and perhaps 2 months' leeway from then to 1½ years of age. If the parents know that children on either side of the family are slow to talk, that information, rather than the milestones indicated in Table 2.1, should form the basis for their expectations. Illness delays development and sometimes results in a temporary setback. Parents should take this into account.

At best, the milestones tell us about "average" children born after a full-term healthy pregnancy. The premature child is likely to be a slow-developing child. This is especially so for the child who is born in the seventh month of pregnancy (or sooner) and who weighs less than 5 pounds. Although we can provide no formula and no schedule for the speech and motor development of premature children, we can provide a rough guide. Allow at least 2 months of postbirth time for each month of prematurity. The best guides can only be provided by a pediatrician, who will assess the child's reflexes and developmental skills. Even then, projections (still only approximate) for the child's future development need to be based on periodic reassessments.

$\mathcal{C}$hapter 3

Early Responses to Voice:
The Voice that Binds and Bonds

Prenatal Responses to Voice?

When does an infant first respond to human voice? Perhaps we might even ask whether the infant-to-be, the fetus in utero, responds to the voice of the mother-to-be? The answer is, "Probably, yes." I have been assured by many mothers that they were able to feel movement months before the child was born when they spoke or sang to the baby-in-waiting. Most of the mothers recall that they addressed the fetus as "baby." A few by a chosen name. Most of the mothers were quite confident that the response to voice was different from that to other noises.[1]

How the infant "learns" to recognize the mother's voice provides support for the view that the capacity for language is an *instinct*. That is, that to be human implies having a brain that is "wired" (patterned) to be receptive and to respond differentially to voice whether or not it is in competition with other noises. The mother's voice, at the outset, is in "competition"

---

[1] On the basis of their own observations and a review of the literature, Klaus and Klaus (1985) stated, "Months before birth, babies' ability to hear is well established." DeCasper and Fifer (1980), using a suckling approach in their study, found that newborns sucked at a rate higher than their usual on hearing a woman's voice, but not a man's. They also found that newborns prefer their mother's voice—presumably heard in utero—to that of other female voices.

with other noises, both internal and external to the developing fetus. Klaus and Klaus (1985, p. 135) asserted:

> From the earliest period of pregnancy, the environment of the womb is a symphony of sounds and vibrations. Minute microphones placed along side the fetus at 6 to 7 months have revealed that the maternal sounds have a volume slightly less that of a busy street! Swishing of the blood in the mother's large blood vessels, her heartbeats, and her intestinal rumblings make up many of the sounds.

Early Infant Responses to Voice

Let us assume that the first voice the new-born child responds to is the mother's. Let us also assume that the response is both instinctive and distinctive.

Nothing is more distinctive in the behavior of infants than their responses to the human voice. Within the first few weeks of life, the baby will respond differently to the voice that purrs and the voice that snarls, to the happy voice and the angry voice. Very early in life, sometimes as early as 3 weeks, the baby may engage in a "dialogue of cooing" with a "cooing" mother. The baby may even learn to wait and take a turn. Angry voices literally "turn babies off." A baby may turn away from the voice or begin to cry. In contrast, the baby is "turned on" and toward the producer of the happy voice, especially if the happy voice is a familiar one. An unexpected voice may produce crying. The sound of the mother's voice may change the crying to cooing and later, when a child is more "sophisticated," to smiles and laughter.

The baby's early responses to the human voice are different from those to any other sounds or noises. We cannot be certain why this is so. It is simply an aspect of what it is to be born a human being. Birds are responsive to other birds' noises, and so singing birds learn to sing. Dogs bark; cats meow; and human beings vocalize and talk. Children who are born with normal equipment are "prewired" to be responsive to human voices. They are also equipped and constructed to make vocal sounds that are expressions of feelings: tender or furious, loving or hateful. They learn to use their voices to cajole or reject, seduce or repel. The voices of human beings can express subtleties beyond the meaning of words. They can even replace words when feelings or meanings cannot be verbalized.

The evolutionist Charles Darwin believed that this very human ability represents "an instinct of sympathy." Beginning in infancy and continuing throughout life, voice is the primary way in which human beings show their feelings and emotions. So the child, with an "instinct of sympathy," is in special tune with other human voices and uses his or her own voice to express feelings and emotions.

Bowlby (1958) considered crying and other forms of infant vocalization to be important attachment behaviors that are highly predictable in the desired outcome of bringing the mother or other caregiver to the child. Later, vocalizations serve to maintain interactions with significant others close to the baby. At a very early age, normal children learn that "dialogues" can be carried on through interchanges of vocalizations.

How is a normal baby likely to vocalize in response to the voice of a person important to caregiving? The investigations of Bruner (1975, 1983), Fernald (1989, 1993), and others, as well as my own observations, suggest that it is possible to make the following generalizations:

- By the end of the first month, the baby cries when exposed to loud noises. The baby may make it a duet when he or she hears another baby crying.

- An adult voice, if it is not an angry voice, will have a soothing (quieting) effect on the baby.

- In the first or second month, the infant responds to a vocalizing adult by smiling. Often the baby will "hold a dialogue" with the adult, "cooing" back to the adult. The baby may restart the "cooing" if the adult stops and so "keep the dialogue going."

- Children will "work" to hear a voice. One investigator, Dr. Sam Rabinovitch (personal communication), measured the energy with which infants as young as 4 weeks suckled on a nipple while they were listening to recordings of their mothers' voices. When the voice recordings were stopped, the babies increased the energy of their suckling until the voices came on again. Then, the suckling energy went back to what was usual for the individual infant.

It is clear that the normal child needs to hear human voice and responds in different ways to what the voice expresses, very early in life. Favorable conditions, such as hearing human voices often, especially ones with soothing qualities, reinforce the infant's natural tendencies to vocalize. Conditions may also reinforce tendencies to be frightened or to be unhappy if the baby's experiences are with unhappy or angry voices. These voices, of course, come from unhappy or angry persons.

The infant, or even the young child, cannot separate the voice from the vocalizer. The two go together in the child's mind, and either the person or the voice will make the child feel happy or afraid, as the case may be. Because children, especially bright children, tend to generalize their responses, they are likely to respond the same way to persons who are like those they already know, that is, respond in kind—with pleasure or displeasure, with joy or apprehension, with anticipation of security and comfort or with fear—to many persons who somehow individually remind them of the first person they associated with a certain feeling or emotion.

The Melody of Speech

"All gone," says mother when the last spoonful of cereal has gone down the hatch. "Upsy baby," she says, when she picks up her baby. Each of these maternal exclamations is spoken with a melody appropriate to the words. Thus "all gone" is uttered as

all gone

and "upsy baby" as

upsy baby

Mother, by her words and appropriate speech "music," is teaching her child that there are patterns of melody that go with the flow of sounds.

Babies can usually distinguish between upward and downward melody (intonation) contours months before they say their first words. So it is no surprise that their own first words are accompanied by melodies that they hear grown-ups speak. Some students of infant speech believe that babies are able to imitate adult speech melodies from 1 to 3 months before they say their first words—well before a year of age. These melodies extend a baby's repertoire beyond simple expressions of feeling and emotion. Preverbal vocal achievements are summarized in Table 3.1.

Table 3.1
Early Vocal Responses and Productions Before First Words

Approximate Age	Baby Hears or Sees	Baby Responds
Birth–2 months	Loud noise	Cries.
	Baby cries	Cries.
	Eye contact with adult	Reflexively yawns, gurgles, coughs, sneezes; coos when content. May produce sounds such as "ayruh" when distressed.
	Angry voice	Baby cries and may turn away from voice.
	Nonangry voice	Coos in response.
2–3 months	Sees face or hears familiar voice	Chuckling noise, laughs.
	Unpleasant voice	Cries.
4–5 months	Social play with adult	Laughs, as for an older child. "Sings," coos when child is alone and content.
6 months	Speaking person	Produces a variety of vocal responses to indicate feelings. May "exclaim" to show delight. Child responds and imitates differences in vocal melody (intonation) patterns.
7–9 months	Presence of familiar person	Child's vocal contours (intonation) suggest requests, demands. Sophisticated cooing expresses calmness and contentment.
10 months or earlier	Adult voice	Child responds by adjusting own pitch level in direction of the voice pitch of the adult, higher when responding to female than to male voice.
12 months	Significant other	Produces increasingly sophisticated vocalizations with communicative intent.

Prospects

The little "tunes" that children learn from their caregivers are preparations for learning intonation—the melody patterns of a language. These patterns become the carriers of our words, from single words such as *no, yes, now, sure,* and *maybe* to phrases and sentences that make sentences and ask questions. These we will consider in our next chapter. As children learn to put words together in a sequence they will later identify as *grammar,* they will also learn to use intonation to be positive and emphatic, negative, doubtful, ironic, sarcastic, angry, and even subtle. They will learn how to express affect, to be able to indicate how they feel about what they think. Some children may indicate this achievement while still using "baby talk" pronunciations. By age 4 years, most children have a minimum of "baby talk" and a rapidly increasing vocabulary. They also have most of the "rules" of grammar under their control. They may reveal this control of grammar by regularizing adult exceptions to grammar by saying *goed* instead of "went"; and "shoozes" instead of "shoes." In time, they will learn the exceptions to rules and so become as unreliable as the adults.

We should not assume that the intonation patterns of English hold for all languages. They do not hold for tonal languages. For a discussion of Asian language and tonal systems, I recommend Cheng's (1991) *Assessing Asian Language Performance.*

$\mathcal{C}$hapter 4

First Sentences

There is something implausible about most views about the acquisition of grammar: whether they be the views of empiricists who think grammar is learned like anything else, or the views of those who claim that there is some sort of innate disposition that fates human beings to be language acquirers. Besides, it seems highly unlikely in the light of our present knowledge that infants learn grammar for its own sake. Its mastery seems always to be instrumental to doing something with words in the real world, if only meaning *is* something.

JEROME BRUNER, *CHILD'S TALK: LEARNING TO USE LANGUAGE*

Next to talking and walking, the concern parents most often express is, "When do we start toilet training our baby?" A pediatrician friend has a standard answer for this query. His answer is, "When your child puts two words together." Once we overheard a parent ask our pediatrician friend, "Why then? How is putting two words together related to toilet training?" We also overheard his answer, "Because before then is too soon. The right time is when your Bobby puts two words together."

I pondered this question for some years, about my own children and in the interests of many other children. The pediatrician was usually right, but why? Now I believe I know the answer. Interestingly, the answer is directly related to the child's stage in language development. This, in turn, is related to the child's general ability to anticipate events.

The Language of Anticipation

In Chapter 2 we left the child using language as commands. Johnny, in addition to labeling, was using his words to get people to do his bidding. Parents may wonder why so often their 15- to 18-month-old child says "toity" or "wuh" (for wet) only after the deed is done. This ability, we may recognize, is just another instance of the child's naming ability. Only when children are able to anticipate *what is about to happen,* when they can both cue and control themselves, can they announce what needs to be done before it is too late. When the child makes a noise—whether it is a grunt or one that sounds like a word—that serves as a signal of what is about to happen, the child also signals that he or she is ready to be toilet trained. In effect, the child is now demonstrating the ability to associate an inner feeling with a consequence, and a consequence with a word. Every parent knows that just because this can be done is no assurance that it will be done, at least regularly. On occasion the child may be too busy with other matters to pay attention to these inner biological happenings. The child may simply not be aware of what is going on, or if aware, may not seem to care. So accidents do and will happen. However, if the rewards are worth the control, accidents become rare, and toilet training is achieved. Parents may take pride in knowing that this control, like speech, is peculiar to human beings.

By the time our Johnny or Mary, our Adam or Eve, can say "baby-toity" or "baby-wuh" (wet) in order to stay clean or dry, he or she usually has a vocabulary of about 50 recognizable words. In addition, the child may have three to five two-word "sentences," and at the same time, is learning to say a great deal with single words. Each word may be used not only to label but to command. A one-word command may have several meanings. In effect, this makes the single word the equivalent of several full statements. For example, cup may simply mean "this thing is called a cup," or possibly "I see that we have a new cup," or "Come now, it's time to fill the cup." How does a parent know which meaning is intended? Only by observing the child's actions and accompanying gestures or early body language.

But it is just as important for the parent to listen to the vocal inflection. Simple naming is likely to be done with a fairly flat vocal inflection, like

$$\longrightarrow$$
cup.

A command to "fill the cup" will have a more imperious downward inflection:

cup.

If the child thinks it may be a cup but you never can tell, the inflection is likely to be rising:

cup.

This is the way speakers of English use voice inflections to make a variety of statements and to ask questions that can ordinarily be answered by a *yes* or *no.*

Creative Listening and Speaking: Combining Words into Sentences

Some children make the most out of these single-word sentences before they combine two or more words into new constructions. By 24 months, most children have begun to use two-word sentences and some have progressed to three words. If your youngster at this age is not yet at this stage but is using single words to indicate a variety of meanings, there is no cause for concern. Suppose, however, that your youngster was a late starter who didn't begin to use recognizable words until 18 months of age. In that case, allow some added time for catching up. A late starter may not begin to use two-word combinations until 30 months of age.

At all times *what is important to notice is whether there is progress in some direction relative to language comprehension or production.* Does the child understand more of what he or she hears? Is the child speaking more of the time, either using more words or suggesting more meanings for the words used? To know for sure, parents need to keep notes and records. They should chart the course of language development over periods of weeks and months rather than days. Somehow, after long enough intervals of time, almost all children achieve approximately the same goal. They understand what you say and, in turn, speak so that you understand them. But each child gets there by a unique and personal route.

The production of *two-word combinations* marks a new and important stage in the child's language development. For most children, this stage usually begins when the child has a vocabulary of at least 50 single-word sentences. A child may achieve this level of development as early as 18 months of age or as late as 30 to 36 months of age. Most children are likely to use two-word combinations by 24 months.

The child uses two-word combinations, just as earlier he or she used single words, for a variety of meanings. For example, *mommy-shoe* may mean "Please, mommy, put on my shoes," "Mommy is putting on my shoes," or "Mommy, put on your shoes so that we can get going." The combination *baby-milk* may mean: "I want milk," "You are about to give me milk," or "I want more milk."

Creative Language and the Use of Syntax

At some time during the two-word-combination stage, most children will begin to say things they have not been specifically "taught." For example, a child who has been "taught" to say "baby up" may, *on his or her own,* say "Daddy up" or "Mommy up."

When children do this they are demonstrating that they learn more than their parents "teach" them. What parents teach a child, or think they have taught, serves as a model. The child uses this model to try out new word combinations. He or she may even reverse the order of the words. Instead of saying "Baby up," the child may try out "Up baby" and "Up dolly" and "Up ball." Now the child has become a creative speaker, and is making it clear not only that he or she understands you but also that this understanding can be generalized. In a very real sense, the child is a generator of new constructions based on models of "old" constructions. Now all that is left in order to become expert in the language game is to build up a vocabulary and learn more about how grown-ups string words together and speak in the breathless way they do.

The period between 18 and 36 months is one of rapid growth in all aspects of language. At 18 months a child may have a speaking vocabulary of about 50 words. By 36 months this vocabulary may increase to 1,000 words or more. Figure 4.1 shows the extremely rapid growth of vocabulary between the ages of 2 and 3 years. Of course, vocabulary growth has no top

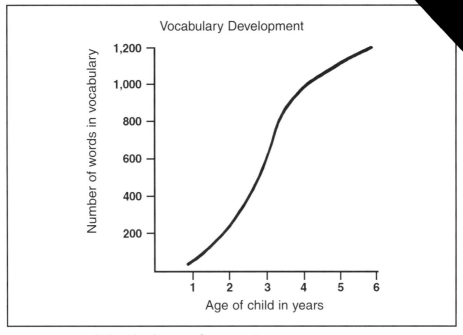

Figure 4.1. Vocabulary development from 1 to 6 years.

age. We continue to learn new words and new meanings of words until we are no longer capable of learning.

By the age of 3 or 4 years, the child's ability to combine words into sentences or other meaningful combinations—that is, to use syntax—closely resembles that of the key adults in his or her special environment. The child's growth in the use of syntax and in pronouncing words clearly parallels a very rapid growth in vocabulary. Except for voice, which happily remains childish, and some "infantile" pronunciations, the child has progressed a long way toward speaking the way adults do.

Learning syntax is a tremendous accomplishment. Yet the child isn't at all aware of how difficult an achievement it is—for children beyond age 10 and for almost all adults. Here are some interesting statistics: However difficult it is for adults to learn a second language, all but 3% to 5% of children learn to speak one or more languages by mere exposure if the exposure is before age 10 years. From ages 10 to 12 it is more difficult to learn a second language and sound like a native speaker. After age 12, second-language learning becomes even more difficult unless a person is completely immersed in the new language and avoids use of the first while establishing the second.

: 3-year-old child, who has already accomplished so
learns how to say things that indicate the present, the
l learns how complicated constructions become that
ı as *if* or *although.* The child also learns what to do
with words to indicate singular or plural and how to change verbs to make
them "agree" with their subject words. Children who speak other languages
may learn that subjects "agree" with predicates not only in number but also
in gender. They learn an amazing number of ways to say complex things in
complex ways. Bilingual children may learn two ways of saying the "same"
thing in two languages. Almost always they learn all these things without
any awareness of the immensity of their achievement. The use of language,
beyond anything else, is what it means to be a human being.

The milestones we have discussed should provide most parents with the
information they need to answer the question, "Is my child progressing normally in speech?" But parents, as well as other persons interested and involved
in the development of the child with mental retardation or deafness, need to
know more.

Children with severe mental retardation, without the benefit of direct,
specific teaching, rarely go beyond the labeling stage in language acquisition. Children with moderate mental retardation are slow in combining
words and slow in reaching the stage where they use conventional (adult)
language constructions. Most, however, do get there. Perhaps when they are
7 or 8 years of age, they are on a 3-year-old level of proficiency. But this is
not too bad. A year or two later they may be almost as good as most 4- or
5-year-olds. By this time, most aspects of grammar are under control. At
least they are able to use and understand sentence constructions like those
used by the adults around them.

Children who are deaf tend to be severely deficient in their use of conventional word constructions. But this may be a reflection of the way they are
taught—or not taught. Authorities on the teaching of the deaf do not agree
on how deaf children should be taught language. Issues between the teaching of oral language or sign language, or new versions of sign language that
incorporate word order and grammatical features of spoken language, are still
much in dispute. In his book *Deafness and Learning* (1973), Furth offered
suggestions as to appropriate instruction for children who are deaf. Although
Furth has had significant influence on the teaching of the deaf, there are still
a variety of views as to how deaf children should be instructed so that their
language and communicative skills will be improved. There is one opinion

on which the profession is unanimous—teaching should begin as early as possible, and age 1 is not too soon! Several controversial issues are reviewed in H. Davis and Silverman (1978), J. M. Davis and Hardick (1981), Eisenson and Ogilvie (1983), and Martin (1986). The writings of Ursula Bellugi are a must! (see, e.g., Bellugi, 1970).

Language Milestones from Age 2 to 4 Years: A Summary

By the age of 2 years, most children have achieved the following:

- They understand hundreds of words and many thousands of sentences that include the words they know.

- They begin to use new combinations based on models or representative sentences that others use. So, now the child who has been "trained" or "taught" a construction such as "Where is the doll?" knows where to look or that he should start looking when he hears, "Where is the doggy?" Similarly, the child who has as her model "Baby-shoe" may herself begin to say "Baby-sock" or "Baby-hat." Children who can do this are creative listeners and creative talkers. They are able to understand things they never heard before and say things they never tried before with full anticipation of being understood.

- The child begins to string words together—that is, to use syntax—like the grown-up speakers in the immediate environment. By 4 years of age, most children are fairly proficient in the use of syntax. By age 5, all but a small percentage of children are almost as proficient as most of the adults in their homes.

From our previous discussion and from Table 4.1, it should be apparent that, for most children, the second birthday marks the start of a dramatic age. It is not only the beginning period of great physical achievement, one when the child develops motor skills and controls, but a period in which we see evidence of rapid intellectual growth. Baby talk begins to give way to more grown-up pronunciations. Within a few months the child may increase his or her speaking vocabulary from 50 words to several hundred. (Note that we are no longer referring to the subject of this book as a "baby" but as a "child.")

Within a year, the youngster's vocabulary may exceed 1,000 words. At age 3 years, the child can speak his or her mind, make intentions clear, and understand an adult's intention, sometimes despite the words the adult may use.

By age 4, except possibly for the sounds *s, th, l,* and *r,* the child is proficient in controlling the sounds of the language. The child's vocabulary continues to grow rapidly, although not at the same rate that it did between the ages of 2 and 4 years. He or she speaks with the syntax of the adults in the surrounding environment. Yet, somehow, the child can speak not only for himself or herself but as a unique self in an individual rhetorical style.

Again, parents should be reminded that these milestones are only approximate guides to accomplishment. Not all children are equally skillful in their physical development. Some are slow in developing their skills, but catch up within 6 months or a year to "normal" or "average" expectation. What we have said of physical skills also holds for speech acquisition. So don't be rigid in your interpretation of the information in Table 4.1. The information is there only to supply approximate guides. If your child deviates too much from the guidelines—say, 6 months or more—discuss the deviation with your pediatrician or family doctor. The doctor should be able to answer your questions, or refer you to another professional person who can. In any event, you have a right to ask and a right to know!

Anticipation, Regulation, and Control

Although Table 4.1 brings us up to age 4, let us concentrate on the highly significant accomplishments in the use of language by most 2-year-olds. At this age, children who have begun to put words together in sentences indicate that they are serious communicators. In their statements, and later in their questions, these 2-year-olds expect something to happen as a consequence of what they say and how they say it. If their expectations are not met, we may be treated to demonstrations of what is meant by "the terrible twos." At this age, we may observe *self-awareness* and *anticipatory awareness*—their anticipations according to their standards of how others are supposed to relate and behave toward them *when they speak!*

Table 4.1

Milestones from 2 to 4 Years

Approximate Age	Child Understands and Says	Child Does
24 months	Understands hundreds of words and sentences. Has a speaking vocabulary of 50 or more words. May begin to use two-word combinations.	Walks with relative ease. Can walk up or down stairs, usually planting both feet on each step before going to next step.
30 months	The child's vocabulary growth is proportionately greater than at any other period. Many, though not all, of the child's sentences are grammatically like those of the adults in his or her life. Understands most of what is said if it is within his or her experience. Articulation (pronunciation) may include some infant sounds, such as *w* for *r*, but almost all of what is said is understood by well-intentioned listeners.	Can jump and stand on one foot. Has good hand and finger coordination. Can build a tower with as many as six blocks.
36 months	Speaking vocabulary may exceed 1,000 words. Syntax almost completely "grown up." Can say what he or she thinks and make intentions clear. Except for voice, the child speaks much as the older members of the community do.	Runs proficiently. Can walk stairs by alternating feet. Hand preference is usually established.
48 months	Except possibly for some difficulty with *s, th, l,* and *r,* the child's articulation (sound production) is under good control. Grammatically, child has acquired much of what he or she is likely to acquire. Yet, somehow, he or she still manages to have a personal style, employing favorite words and individual ways of turning a phrase. Has an individual "rhetorical" style.	Can hop on one foot, usually the right one unless left-handed. Can throw a ball in the direction of an intended receiver. Can catch a ball in arms and occasionally with both hands. Can walk on a line. Is able to ride a tricycle and perhaps a small bicycle.

Halliday (1975) classified the communicative efforts of 2-year-olds into three broad categories: interaction, regulation, and personal control. These communicative categories serve seven functions:

1. *Instrumental*—language used to satisfy specific material needs: "I [me] want kitty," "I want cookie," "I want [something material]."

2. *Regulatory*—language to exert control or direct the behavior of another person: "Daddy come," "Mommy up."

3. *Interactional (social gesture)*—language used to establish or maintain contact with an important other person; for example, "Please, mommy," "Hi, gamma."

4. *Heuristic*—language used to investigate or explore the environment: "There doggy," "What that?"

5. *Personal*—language to announce and express individuality, to speak of oneself; for example, "I [me] girl," "I [me] jump," "I pretty."

6. *Imaginative*—language used in make-believe play or to create a pretend world; for example, "I'm a doggy," "I'm a mommy," or even, if the need arises, "Me baby."

7. *Informative*—in contrast to the heuristic, language employed to provide information, real or imaginary, to someone who is elected to hear it. This use of language may overlap the factual; for example, "I'm a big bear" is both imaginative and informative, whereas "Puffy is my kitty" may be factual but not imaginative.

It is obvious that some of the functions of language overlap. For example, "I'm a big bear" may inform a listener of her expected role in a game in which the child announces an intended action. "I run" or "I jump" also serves as a regulator of an intended action.

Chapter 5

How Can I Help My Child Express Thoughts?

"Look, mommy, I caught a pretty butterfly." Four-year-old Susie, full of excitement, is showing mother her prize catch. "Yes, dear, it's pretty," her mother confirms.

"Look, mommy, I caught a pretty butterfly." An equally excited 4-year-old José is showing mother his prize catch. "Uh, huh," his mother acknowledges, "Run along and play."

What has the mother told her child in each of these "conversations?" Susie received confirmation that the butterfly was pretty. Perhaps that is all Susie expected. She may have wanted to show her prize to several other persons important to her. Indeed, if her posture suggested that she barely had time to stop, that she was poised to keep going, mother said just enough. What did little José get from his mother? At best, begrudging acknowledgment that her child had said something to her. But no confirmation about what he said or showed his mother. The "Run along and play" was a more or less polite dismissal, a way of indicating that she had no wish for further talk with her child.

Now let's take a third example of a child and mother interchange. "Look, mommy, I caught a pretty butterfly." An excited little Mary is looking expectantly at her mother.

"Yes, dear, it's pretty," her mother answers. Then, noting that Mary is "at rest" and not "on the wing," she adds, "Can you see the four powdery wings?"

Now our child and mother have an opportunity for enriching the meaning of *butterfly*. Mary's attention is directed to the fact that butterflies have four wings and that the wings are covered with a powdery substance. Mary might ask now, "What is powder?" or possibly observe, "Birds have two wings, but butterflies have four." So Mary's concept of a butterfly is enriched. Beyond this, Mary also appreciates that mother enjoys talking to her and perhaps knows a thing or two worth listening to and learning.

Mary's mother did not overwhelm her child by offering the information that butterflies are members of the insect class *lepidoptera,* that the class includes moths, butterflies, and skippers, or that skippers are closely related to but are not true butterflies. Unless a little Mary or José is extremely precocious, such information would be gratuitous and confusing.

Instead, note how fortunate little Mary is in the responses she received from her mother. She learned that her mother really listens to her and that speaking is a reliable, fruitful, and potent mode of behavior. Children who have parents who respond as Mary's did learn that they are significant members of their families, that their feelings and their thinking, their observations and discoveries, really matter and can be shared. Through such responses and relationships, children mature intellectually and emotionally.

Shaping the Structures of Language: What a Parent Can Do

What can parents do to help their children acquire and develop good language skills? The most general and most significant answer is: *Provide a good example.* A good example includes an overall family setting in which adults listen to one another and to children. The setting is one in which statements and questions are understood for their real intent, and not for their literal meanings. A good setting also includes some direct talking in well-constructed sentences to younger children, especially those below age 3 years.

Some children are ultimately more proficient than others. Vocabulary growth and development may continue throughout life. But even as children, some persons are considerably more proficient than others. In part, proficiency is related to mental capacity. By and large, bright children are ahead of normal children, who are ahead of dull normal children in their potential for language proficiency. But a few special human beings have a flair for language. They can just speak and write better than most of us.

Four-year-olds are usually well along in their language acquisition. They are likely to use the grammatical structures of adults; they have a productive vocabulary of between 1,500 and 2,000 words; and they understand up to 20,000 words that they hear. With good models and satisfactory experience, motivated children can be left to their caring environments to mature in their verbal behavior. Yet, great as are the achievements of most 4-year-olds, the linguistic accomplishments of children from 2 to 3 years of age are even more impressive.

Some 2-year-olds are just beginning to speak. Their speaking vocabularies may not exceed 50 words. At age 3 years, most children have speaking vocabularies of 1,000 or more words. Two-year-olds are just beginning to use two-word combinations. By 3, most children can say what they are thinking, using sentence structures that are essentially the same as those of the key adults in their environments.

So it is in the "galloping" age between 2 and 3 that parents can play roles and take responsibility for shaping the language habits and attitudes of their children. Most parents, we hasten to say, need no urging to do what is needed for their children. What they do intuitively is usually correct and beneficial.

Nevertheless, just in case, we will make some observations and suggestions. We begin with a 2-year-old, or any child, regardless of age, who is just beginning to put two words together for some first "sentences." We have three goals in mind. The first is to assure the child that we are listening. The second is to understand the child's intended meaning. The third is to provide a more grown-up construction as a model for the child without rejecting what the child has offered. Here are several minidialogues.

CHILD: Dolly chair.

PARENT: Yes, dolly is in the chair.

CHILD: Baby milk.

PARENT: Baby drinks her milk.

CHILD: Boy jump.

PARENT: The boy is jumping.

CHILD: Boy shoe.

PARENT: It's the boy's shoe.

CHILD: No boy's shoe.

PARENT: Boy puts on his shoe.

CHILD: Boy shoe.

PARENT: Yes, the boy puts on his shoe.

In the first three minidialogues, the parent guessed the intended meaning of the child's utterance. In each instance, the parent expanded the child's verbal production by adding verb forms and one or more functional words (prepositions, articles) so that it became an adult-type sentence. But note that even though the child's sentences were modified, the parent kept the original (that is, the child's) word order. The parent preserved what the child said, accepting it rather than rejecting it.

In the fourth minidialogue, the parent did not at once guess the child's meaning. "Boy shoe" may mean a number of things, depending on the circumstances. This child's sentence might mean "The boy has a [one] shoe," "The boy is looking for his shoe," "The boy found his shoe," or "The boy is putting on [or taking off] his shoe." And we haven't even exhausted all possible meanings. The sentence might even mean "The boy has no shoe." Often, parent and child must play a guessing game as to the child's intended meaning. Watching the child closely, but not anxiously, and observing whether the child is pointing to some detail may help in the guessing game and bring the dialogue to a satisfactory conclusion. Each restatement offered by the adult is a guess—a well-educated guess, we hope—as to what the child may mean.

The guess, in adult construction form, is an expression of meaning. Even if the parent guessed wrong, the child is exposed to a possible meaning the sentence may have, and to a way of expressing that meaning. The child learns from all of these restatements of his or her own utterances.

Now, let's look at another device that will provide the child with an opportunity to acquire meanings and vocabulary. Again, here are several minidialogues:

CHILD: Kitty purr.

PARENT: Yes, the kitty is happy.

CHILD: Tree moves.

PARENT: The wind is bending the tree.

CHILD: Baby cry.

PARENT: The baby is hungry.

How are these minidialogues different from those presented earlier? In each instance, the parent has added something to what the child said, offering new key words that spell out new meanings. In the first interchange, the child has an opportunity to learn that the word *purr* is associated with a happy state for a kitty. In the second interchange, the child learns that the wind makes the tree bend. In the third instance, the child is offered a possible and likely cause for a baby's crying.

Although these interchanges do not include all of the child's original words, some of them are retained. Meanings are more broadly expanded than in the earlier minidialogues. In fact, these interchanges follow the suggestion of developmental psychologists, including myself and Peter and Jill de Villiers (1979, pp. 46–48): The child is offered additional meanings, stated in adult form, at a time when the child is most likely to be attentive to what the adult has to say.

We should note also that the child has not been overwhelmed with too many meanings or too many words. Nor did the child's offering become a point of departure for philosophical explanations or little essays by the adult. The matter of keeping the dialogue open and going is left to the child. That is how it should be when a child begins an interchange.

Verbal Constriction

So far in this chapter, and for most of the book, we have accentuated the normal and the positive. Now we will direct attention to the negative, specifically to a form of verbal behavior that happens all too often when a child is talking to a parent or other adult who is important to the child.

Bobby, full of age-3 excitement, has just rushed in from the garden to present his prize, or at least share it, with his mother. "Looky, mommy, I found a wriggly thing." Bobby's mother, taken by surprise and unable to conceal her feelings, responds, "Bobby, throw that dirty worm away and go wash your hands."

Now, what has Bobby learned? At most, that the wriggly thing is called a "worm." It may, of course, not have been a worm at all, but a caterpillar. Bobby's mother was too concerned with her own aversion to worms to take time to look. She did take time to describe the wriggly thing as dirty and so ordered Bobby to go wash his hands. What the child probably learned is that it is unwise to share discoveries with his mother. If he does, he may have to wash his hands at an off time not in any way related to meals or company coming. Above all, Bobby has probably learned that it is sometimes safer to keep quiet than to talk.

What might Bobby have learned if his mother responded directly rather than *tangentially,* or indirectly, to his words and discovery? He might have learned why worms are a bit dirty, or that this particular wriggly thing was a caterpillar rather than a worm. All of this, and possibly much more, might have been Bobby's if his mother had responded directly rather than tangentially. With a little bit of acting, the mother might have shared in discovery and expanded her son's acquisition of meanings. Instead, probably unintentionally, the mother created a groundwork for anxiety about communication. Perhaps, even worse, Bobby may learn to become that kind of communicator himself.

The Development of Concepts

Concepts Without Words: The Infant

It is a rare parent who has not learned that babies become attached to toys. Substituting a new toy for an old one, however similar they may seem to the adult, may become a traumatic household experience. When the infant is given a first doll, it is held and smelled and tasted. It is felt and manipulated. Thus, the doll is experienced through all of the baby's senses. The sum total of the experiences constitutes the doll. If in time the first doll is so worn out (from the adult's point of view) as to justify replacing it, the cautious parent offers a second doll but does not remove the first. It is up to the infant to decide whether the second—doll, ball, rattle, or whatever—is satisfactory. If it is, the adult may assume that the child's standards for that particular toy have been met. Doll No. 2 may not be exactly like Doll No. 1, but it will do!

Many babies put their households into a state of uproar when it is time to introduce a new item into the young one's diet. When at last cereal or spinach is accepted in infant food form, each spoonful of cereal, or liquidy spinach, or syrupy apricot must have the same consistency and texture as every other spoonful. Anticipations (expectations and concepts) must be met, or else!

Fortunately, there are a few infants who are able to accept minor differences in toys and foods, so that the households are not in recurrent or even chronic states of anxiety. These infants, even before they can speak their needs, seem to have fairly flexible concepts. If things are essentially the same, the baby accepts them.

These examples show that normal babies have a number of "concepts" (ideas) in the first months of their lives. In fact, they have concepts from 6 months to a year or more before they have words.

Concepts, Language, and Meaning

What does a 2-year-old mean by the words "Pitty titty" (pretty kitty) when looking at the household pet? The child may mean a number of things, have a number of things in mind. The child may mean no more than "I see the kitten," "I want the kitten I see," "I like the kitten," "Bring the kitten closer to me," or "I want to hold or stroke the kitten." Each of these meanings is not mutually exclusive of the other. But one thing is certain. The child has a name for the domesticated animal. The name incorporates the child's experience with this member of the household. If the child does not produce a pronunciation of "pretty kitty" unless the animal is in view, then we may conclude that *not in sight is not in mind.* The child needs actual sensory experience to evoke the name.

However, most 2-year-olds are not dependent upon immediate and full objective experience to have things in mind. A picture of a kitten will evoke the name. The sound of a cat's meowing or purring or even lapping up milk may also evoke the name. When this occurs, the child has arrived at an important stage in intellectual (cognitive) development. A special aspect (attribute) of the behavior of a pet has the power to evoke a response initially made to the real event. Soon the name of the thing or event, such as "pretty kitty" can become a "stand-in." That is, it can stand for the real thing.

Later in the child's experiences and intellectual development, he or she may learn that not all cats, not even all domestic cats, meow or purr and that not all cats live in homes or sleep in protected places provided by human beings in their households. The child will learn that certain ideas—his or her concepts—require modification and revision: There are broad categories and subcategories and confusing categories. But, if the child is a good learner, he or she will also learn what differences are important in categorizing and naming various things and events.

The child, usually without knowing just how, will begin to appreciate that having names for things and happenings helps to establish distinctions and develop concepts. The child will also learn that having many word names for objects and actions is helpful in effectively sharing ideas. So, as the child matures, he or she will call some cats Persians and others Angoras and still others Calicos. The child growing up also learns that animals such as lions, tigers, bobcats, jaguars, leopards, and lynx are also cats.

Ultimately, when the child is fairly well grown up, a different kind of knowledge comes. It is the knowledge that adults use some words without any reference to the word's literal meaning. "Catty" is a derogative term rarely if ever applied to biological felines. About the same time, the child learns that though some adults have no objection to being called "kittens," they are likely to have great objection to being called "cats." How the child learns this kind of distinction is beyond the purpose of this book. We will content ourselves with considering how a child develops concepts, and the role of the parent in establishing concepts and conceptual thinking.

The Refinement of Meaning: Generalization and Specialization

When can a parent know that a child has formed a general concept—that is, has generalized experience beyond the mere naming of a particular experience? One signal is when the word *mommy* or *daddy* no longer exclusively designates one of the child's very own relatives. However embarrassing it may be when a child whose father has a moustache commits the "error" of calling any moustached adult "daddy," we can assume that the child has the capacity for generalization. Of course, it is not likely that "daddy," as the label for a moustached man, designates a child–adult relationship. The name may have application only to the single feature *moustache* for an adult. Either way, however, we have an indication of generalization—in fact, of over-generalization in the adult sense.

Similarly, we have evidence of generalization when a child refers to all four-legged animals as "cats," "dogs," or "horses," depending upon the child's first experiences with these animals. Be it a moustache or four legs, what the child tells us by the use of a name is that, on the basis of personal experiences, a particular common feature has emerged. Despite differences the child may or may not overlook, he or she considers the common feature to be the one that defines the category. If the child were the philosopher or psychologist he or she may later become, this thinking could be verbalized by stating, "One of the essential conditions for the formation of a concept is to have a number of experiences that are similar in one or more respects. The individual's recollected responses to the cluster or constellation of experiences is the concept."

It becomes clear, then, that to help a child develop concepts, we need to provide a series of experiences (events or objects) that have many similar features. We show the child several kittens or pictures of kittens, several apples, several babies, several birds, and so on. When the child is provided with a name that encompasses each set of experiences, then we have a conceptual word. So, embarrassment may be avoided, or at least not repeated, if the child has the word *man* rather than *daddy* for an adult with a moustache. Later, when the child becomes aware of incidental (nonessential) features and learns the names for these features, we can help the child express modified concepts in phrases such as "man with moustache," "woman with red hair," "black kitty," "white duck," and so on.

Now, how about the opposite of generalization? How does a child learn that though two animals (a broad concept) have four legs each, one is a dog and one is a cat? If the child has both animals in the home, or opportunities for direct experiences with both of these domesticated creatures, the names he or she hears for them may help. If the dog is called Fido and the cat Felicia, the child may generalize these names to all dogs and all cats. If the cat is called "kitty" and the dog "doggie," then these names will be associated with the animals in more stable ways. The child is likely to learn that kitties are different from doggies and later that cats are different from dogs.

We do not need to have the real things in our homes to highlight differences that make differences as well as similarities that are essential in the formation of concepts. Toys with characteristic features and pictures will do. Later, by the time the child is of school age, even words will do. In the child's early experiences, however, the greater the number of direct and actual experiences the better. With such experiences, not overlooking those made available by books and television, children's concepts can be broadened as well as sharpened. So a child may go not only from *kitty* to *cat* to *tiger,* but also to *animal.* Such learning—the development and modification of concepts—continues throughout life. For the fortunate child, such learning begins in the crib.

Chapter 6

Questions and Cognitive Development

Why Do Children Ask Questions?

What purposes do questions serve? Why, once they get started, do most children ask so many questions? A general answer is that children ask questions because, through the answers they receive, they can get more and learn more than they could if they didn't ask questions. At first, they want to obtain things and information about things. Later, children use questions to get information to satisfy their intellectual curiosity as well.

When children are infants, parents anticipate most of their needs. As their minds mature, they begin to have needs that, fortunately, cannot be readily anticipated. These needs go beyond physical comfort and security. They need to know for the sake of knowing! First questions may, however, be deceiving. When the child asks, "Doddy (dolly)?" or "What dat (that)?" he or she is probably trying to obtain something, rather than learn something. First questions may simply indicate that the child has discovered a new tool or technique to serve an old purpose. Thus, first questions are usually new ways with words that permit children to satisfy their needs. Later, the same device and the very same words may be used to gain information related both to earlier needs and to new ones.

Children's questions reveal that something is going on in their minds that can be satisfied only with the help of others. Presumably, these others

are more skillful or have longer reaches or particular possessions that interest children. So children put other persons to work for them. In doing so,
they become socialized. They use questions, even those used for obtaining
physical things, to involve the persons around them in some kind of social
cooperation. Through questions, inexperienced children make use of the
experience, abilities, and knowledge of adults.

First Questions and
Their Cognitive Significance

Eighteen-month-old Terrence asks, "Cookie?" and indicates that he wants
somebody to give him a little cake. The inflection of his voice, if Terrence is
an English-speaking child, will follow this contour:

cookie.

In asking for his goodie with a single word and an upward inflection, Terrence expects, or at least hopes, that the answer will be "yes." Further, he
expects that appropriate action will accompany or follow the verbal response.
The answer might be "no," of course, but it is unlikely that a wise Terrence
will ask for something that might be denied. If Terrence is not allowed to
have the cookie, he may resort to an old and usually successful mode of
behavior—and achieve by crying what he failed to obtain by talking.

At 18 months, the child is likely to ask questions only about things in
sight, things heard, or at least things he or she can touch. The typical 18-
month-old child is still pretty much tied to the here and now, to responding and dealing with matters that are part of his or her immediate experience. These experiences, literally, are ones that the child can touch, smell,
and see. So the question "Cookie?" is likely to occur only when a cookie is
present and in view but not in the child's reach. At a later stage in cognitive
development, the child may use the same single-word form to ask questions
about matters not in sight, to get answers to little puzzling thoughts such as
"Later?" or "Now?"

At 18 months, most children reach a two- to three-word language stage,
at which they begin to combine words in statements such as "Tom ball,"
"John cookie," and "Kitty eat." Some of the children progress rapidly from

two-word statements to longer ones, such as "Ride in wagon," or even "I [me] ride in wagon." We may also hear children's observations about what other children or grown-ups are doing, such as "Boy throwing ball" and "Man riding bike."

About the time when children begin to produce two- and three-word statements, they also ask their first questions that begin with interrogative (question) words. The first of these interrogative words is likely to be *where* or *what.* Usually, but by no means invariably, the future order of development for interrogative words is *who, why, how,* and *when.* Together, despite the spelling of *how,* sentences that start with interrogative words are called *wh-* questions.

Except for the onset of talking, there is no better indicator that all is going well in the mental development of the child than the ability to understand and ask questions. Through questions, especially those that go beyond *yes* and *no* for answers, children reveal that their minds have the capacity to deal with matters that are not physically present. With the *wh-* questions (*where, who, what, why, how,* and *when*), the child's mind can roam and range through time and space.

Now the child can talk and think about what happened during some yesterday, however vague that yesterday may be. The child can talk and speculate about tomorrow. Questions and questioning that began as devices for getting things done soon advance to devices for exercising imagination and testing thinking. These uses of questions should assure parents that all is going well with the child.

Different Kinds of Yes/No Questions

The earliest questions that children ask are usually designed to bring a *yes* or *no* answer—hopefully, a *yes* response. As they grow, children discover several different ways of phrasing these *yes/no* questions.

Typically, in early stages, the word order of a question takes the form of a statement: "Cookie?" or "Mommy cookie?" Later, the question may be elaborated to "May I have a cookie?" The rising vocal inflection at the end of the "statement" as well as the overall structure of the utterance indicates that this is in fact a question.

The question "Dolly?" may be a polite command. The child knows that, although he or she is asking a question, you know that you are expected to comply as if it were a request, "Please hand me my dolly." This kind of question may be a forerunner of the adult question, "Would it trouble you to close the door?" If the answer is "No trouble at all," without any move to close the door, then the listener either didn't understand the first speaker's intention or preferred to pretend that he or she didn't understand it.

"Is dolly sleeping?" is a second form of the *yes/no* question. Now the child has learned that questions can be asked by changing the order of the words from a statement structure, as in "Dolly is sleeping," to one that begins with the verb. No matter what inflection the child uses, this form of question requires a response from a listener.

A third way to ask a *yes/no* question is to present the order of the words as a statement and then to tag on a *huh* or the equivalent. So we may have "The boy [is] running, huh?" The *huh* is a rough equivalent of the adult forms, *Right?* or *Yes?* or *No?* or *Isn't it?* or *Can't I?* By age 5 years, most children can understand as well as produce such questions.

As children learn the variety of ways to get a *yes* or *no* answer, they use the rising inflectional form alone much less often. But, as most adults know, children do not abandon this first way of asking questions. They simply acquire other ways, which they employ according to circumstances, their needs, and their developing styles. Thus a 6-year-old's request for a piece of candy may take several forms:

- To a friend, also age 6 years: "Got one for me, huh?"

- To an adult, other than a parent: "Please, may I have a piece of candy?"

- To a parent, if the relationship is informal and cordial: "Could I have a piece of candy?" or just "Candy?"

(What would the relationship be if a 6-year-old asks a parent, "Please, I would like a candy?")

Interrogative Word Questions: *Wh-* and *How*

Where

"*Where* boy run?" "*Where* that?" "*Where* mommy going?" These are examples of early *where* questions. In 2 or 3 months, the child may ask the same question in a more complete grammatical form, such as "Where is the boy running?" or "Where is that?" or even "Where is daddy going?" The child expects that the answer will be a location word or phrase. So, whether it is "Where boy run?" or "Where is the boy running?" an answer such as "To his house" or "To the store" is appropriate.

A little later in the child's career, a location word answer may not be enough. The child may continue the questioning by asking "Why?" We will not pretend to have an adequate answer to *why* questions, which we discuss again a little later. Caregivers will have to figure out these answers according to their own intellectual resources. Children who are acquisitive need to be inquisitive (that is, children who are acquiring language need to ask questions) and older persons are supposed to fall in line by providing answers. *What* and *where* questions are usually easy to answer. *Why* questions are a challenge to intellect, imagination, and endurance. For whatever comfort it may provide to caregivers, the number of questions that begin with *why* increases with the child's age, intellectual development, and language proficiency.

Who

Who, the child somehow learns, is reserved for persons and respected animals. He or she may begin to use *who* even before adult forms of the question are mastered. So we may get "Who that?" or, more likely, "Who dat?" several months before "Who is that?" The question form *who* may be used by the child to engage a parent in conversation. For example, a child may point to a girl or a boy in a picture and ask the parent, "Who is throwing ball?" or point to a baby and ask, "Who is sleeping?" If the parent answers appropriately, the child may keep the game going of I Point and Ask and You Tell. Lucky parents usually have a turn to ask questions and to approve of their child's answers. Later, *who* questions may take the more adult form of "Who is eating the candy?" or "Who is driving the car?" or "Who is the girl helping?"[1]

---

[1] The subtle distinction between *who* and *whom* (the subject word and the object word in formal, "old-fashioned" grammar) is likely to escape even the most inquisitive child for many years. Early use is almost always limited to *who* as the subject or object in the sentence.

What

What questions come early in the child's career as a speaker. Most children ask, "What dat [that]?" shortly after they begin to put two words together in a single utterance. "What dat?" may be a real question or a pseudo-question. In fact, *what* is likely to be used simply to engage an adult in conversation before it is used to obtain information. Even then it is interesting to note that the child is asking for a name and so perhaps may be going through a second naming stage. This time, however, the child is getting someone else to supply the names of things.

As the child develops a sense of grammar, the form of the *what* questions is likely to be close to that of an adult's. Then we may hear, "What is that?" and "What is mommy carrying?" The child is still asking that something be named. Soon, however, the child may ask that events and actions be named, as in "What boy do?" and, later, the adult form, "What is the boy doing?" and "What is the girl [or mommy or daddy] reading?" Often, we suspect, children ask *what* questions to make sure of certain names and information rather than to obtain new names or new information. The parent should play along with the child in this "game," even when the parent knows that the child knows and the child knows that the parent knows. Children as well as adults have a right to ask rhetorical and pretend questions, as well as genuine information-seeking questions.

What if questions are a long leap in mental development from the *what* questions, even though the child advances to them rather soon after framing the first *what* questions. When the child asks questions like "*What if* it rains?" or "*What if* daddy comes late?" the parent knows that the child can now deal with future and uncertain events, with abstractions. *What if* questions keep parents sharp in their thinking and in their intellectual resources—a very good state of affairs for all members of a family.

Why

As most parents of 2-year-olds have learned, there is no limit to the number of situations about which children ask *why*. Children, if they are on the precocious side, begin to ask about the *why* of matters as early as 18 months. Some of the *why* questions may be perplexing to adults because the answers lie within the child's own experience. Here is an actual dialogue between a mother and a 20-month-old child:

CHILD: Why me pill [spill] milk?

MOTHER: You were not looking.

CHILD: Why me not looking?

We suspect that if there was an answer to this child's question, only the child could provide it. However, it is likely that the child was engaging in social dialogue, perhaps to divert the mother's attention from the minor but recurrent catastrophe of milk spilling.

Children Who Ask Few Questions

Some children are slow to begin to ask questions, and continue to ask relatively few questions after they have begun. My investigations indicate that there are three groups of children like this.

The first group consists of children who are either ignored or rejected. The rejection may take the form of a thoughtless and unreasonable "No," or a response in the form of "Don't ask so many questions." Parents who are guilty of either the unreasoned "No" or the discouraging "Don't ask . . ." might ask themselves the following:

- What does a child need to do to get *yes* for an answer?

- How many questions would not be too many?

- What should the child do as a substitute for asking questions? (This may be the most important question of all.)

If these questions are answered honestly, most parents will discover that they want their children to continue with the questions, and that they are willing to begin providing answers.

A second group of children who ask few questions and begin to ask them rather late in their careers are those who are slow in mental development. Interestingly, however, the order of questions these children ask parallels that of normal and bright children.

A third group of children who are both slow starters and reluctant questioners, but not intellectually retarded, are ones who are severely delayed in language acquisition. This is a very special but small group of children, some of whom are brain damaged, who are very slow in speech development.

Some of them may not have spoken their first words until age 4 or 5 years. Many of them appear to be unable to learn to speak by means of normal exposure to speaking adults. They need to be directly taught because of their severe limitation for learning and acquiring language by exposure.

This very special group is the subject of the book *Aphasia and Related Disorders in Children* (Eisenson, 1984). I have studied more than 100 of these children and discovered that even at ages 9 and 10 years, when they have overcome most of their language delay, they still seem disinclined to ask questions. This is both surprising and perplexing because, even after they have demonstrated that they do comprehend questions of all types and on occasion can use question constructions, they are much less likely to do so, compared with younger children on the same level of language development. A possible explanation for this apparent disinclination is that the use of the interrogative implies an ability and willingness to deal with the abstract. Aphasic children, as a total population, are more concrete minded and more inclined to deal with the here and now, with objective realities, that do not ordinarily require the use of question constructions. This conjecture would particularly hold for *why, when,* and *how* words in *wh-* questions.

Alternative Strategies to Asking Questions

Are children who ask few questions necessarily those who are or were delayed in language development? Not at all, if there is no other indication of language delay and especially if the child has effective strategies to get answers and actions without having to ask questions. My granddaughter, for reasons I was not able to discern, asked very few questions at an age when most of her peers had discovered the wonder of *wh-* words. Although she asked few questions, she was able to get many answers. Her strategy might be identified as positive thinking. For instance, if she wanted to visit a friend or favorite relative, she was likely to say to her parents, "Tomorrow, let's go visit David." This manner of indicating her wish often resulted in a fairly lengthy dialogue, which she expected and in which she held her own. (As a grandparent I might note that she began holding her own moments after she was born.) By age 3 years, sharpened and motivated by competition with her 6-year-old brother, she was not only highly proficient in language but also fully able to protect her rights and privileges through actions as well as words. At bedtime, my granddaughter collected her books and then addressed a selected, privileged relative with "It's story reading time." As an admiring but still objective observer, it was clear that although this granddaughter did not resort to questions, neither did she entertain any doubt that her statement (invitation) would produce the action she expected to follow.

As with older children and adults, asking a question may frequently be a way of opening a dialogue, a social interchange with another potential speaker. The answer, whether it is a direct response to the question, indicates a willingness to continue the dialogue. Children learn this use of "questions" by observing adults play this social-verbal game.

There are many young granddaughters and grandsons who ask questions—especially *why, how,* and *when* questions—perhaps more often than most children. *What if* questions may occur more often than the simple *what.* For reasons that are only subjective and personal, I consider to be on the bright side both those children who can and do ask questions and those who use alternative strategies for getting the answers and the actions they want. In this respect, children who frequently or occasionally use alternative strategies fulfill the two basic functions served by questions.

Initially, questions are social tools. Through asking questions, children get other persons involved in the satisfaction of their needs. At first, these needs are usually actions that cannot be accomplished alone by the questioner, because the cookie or the friend or the relative is beyond easy reach. Later, the child may seek information, or want confirmation of what he or she already knows, from an esteemed listener. Finally, children seek explanations as well as information and confirmation. They may, of course, still be making sure of their own observations and explanations. Questions and still more questions, or alternative strategies for asking questions, are expressions of maturing minds. The answers children receive are the reflections of maturing adults.

Questions in Form but Not Intent

"Why don't you close the door when you come in?" "Do you mind turning down the radio?" "How many times must I ask you to wash your hands before you eat?" These are examples of pseudo-questions that the young child is typically exposed to; the child learns that these do not really call for answers that inform, explain, affirm, or negate. What the child learns also is to appreciate the intended rather than the literal meaning of a message. In these instances, the message is presented in the form and disguise of a question.

When an adult asks a child, "Is this a green or red ball?" the likelihood is that, unless the questioner is color blind, the purpose of the "question" is not a request for information but rather a way to determine a child's knowledge of red and green. Sometimes it is used to teach these colors. This form of "questioning" may also be used to show off a child's knowledge to another person, who is to be impressed.

Although young children are not likely to use these pseudo-questions in self-initiated dialogues with adults, they may and do use them in play with their peers or their dolls or stuffed animals and sometimes with their live pets, who are not expected to respond.

Later Questions

Between ages 3 and 4 years, children are able to ask questions that include a negative word in the interrogative form. Examples are "Can't Bobby play?" "Why won't Bobby play?" "Won't we go to the park?" or "Why don't we eat now?" These are sophisticated forms of questions that reveal an ability to employ complex grammatical constructions. When children are able to ask such questions, they are also able to construct such complex sentences as "Mommy feeds the baby who is hungry" and "Mary drinks the juice because she is thirsty." They may also appreciate the subtle distinction between "Do you want to go?" and "Don't you want to go?" In summary, children use questions or strategies to avoid possible *no* answers to some questions, to reveal their thinking. They also reveal that their thinking is no longer restricted to the here and now. Early questions, like early statements, reflect needs for names or children's desires for getting someone to do something they cannot do for themselves. Their questions—or perhaps the process of questioning—permit a delay in action and the involvement of another person in a contemplated action. Later questions (questioning) may be used to make sure of certain information or to gather information and opinion as to the *whys, why nots*, and *hows* of what is happening in a world bounded only by the child's imagination.

Children also learn that things are not always what they seem to be, in the way adults use question constructions for a variety of purposes that are a far cry from the first questions addressed to or asked by them. What they are learning is related to the pragmatics of language usage—how to say what you need to say to enhance the likelihood that your message will be understood and you will get what you want.

Chapter 7

Is My Child Speaking Distinctly?
The Selected Sounds for Speech

hen children are at the babbling stage of sound making, they are universalists in their production. They produce sounds in babble play that, by chance, include ones of their native language-to-be. Some of the sounds made in their oral play may not be present in any known language, but these will soon drop out to make good on the promise that the instinct for language allows for selectivity, and soon, in children's echolalic stage, there sounds are so much like the speech sounds of those about them that they seem to be speaking.

When children begin to put sounds into words that are intended to communicate meaning, they start all over again on a selection of sounds—both single ones and combinations—that are identified as words, even though what the words are may escape the decoding ability of members of the family. In effect, the child is engaged in serious baby talk.

The sounds of baby talk are not random products. Almost always, the earliest speech sounds include *m*, *n*, *d*, *b*, *g*, and possibly *p*. This enables the child to say "mamma," "dadda," "doddy," and something like "nah" as a negative. Table 7.1 provides us with a guide for the usual—but by no means invariable—sequence of speech sound acquisition. But do note that all age dates are approximate. By age 7 or 8 most children have the speech sounds of their language under control.

Table 7.1

Approximate Average Age (in Years)
of Control of Consonant Sounds[a]

Average Age	Consonant Sounds
2	*h, m, n, w, b, p, t, k, g, ng, d*
3	*f, y, s, r, l*
4	*ch, sh, j, z, v*
5	*th* (*think*), *th* (*that*)
6	*zh* (*azure*)

Note. Adapted from "When Are Speech Sounds Learned?" by E. K. Sander, 1972, *Journal of Speech and Hearing Disorders, 37,* p. 62.

[a]Vowel sounds are learned early in the child's selection of speech sounds. Unless the child has a severe hearing loss or an uncorrected cleft palate, we take the control of vowel sounds for granted.

How Distinct Should a Child's Speech Be?

"Is my child speaking distinctly?" When parents ask this question, they may suspect that the answer will be "no." But typical childish speech is no cause for concern. Remember the biblical observation from Corinthians? "When I was a child, I spoke as a child, I understood as a child, I thought as a child; but when I became a man, I put away childish things."

A child is entitled to have childish, even infantile, speech. Not until children are 7 or 8 years of age can we expect most of them to have put aside childish speech (if not childish thoughts). Then, except for vocal pitch and "quality," they do in fact speak like adults.

Another answer to "How distinct should a child's speech be?" is "Distinct enough so that the child's messages are intelligible." Intelligibility—how easily a message can be understood—depends on many things, including the listener. Fathers often have a more difficult time understanding (decoding) the speech of their children than mothers do. Older children frequently do much better than either parent. In fact, in some families, big brothers and sisters are the official interpreters for the household.

Speech should become more distinct, of course, as the child grows older. Speech that is distinct enough (decodable) for a 12- to 18-month-old child is "below standard of acceptability" for a 2-year-old. What we find acceptable for a 2-year-old is in turn below what we expect for a 3-year-old.

Distinctness in speech depends on several factors:

1. *Articulation*—production of the sounds of a given language system.
2. *Pronunciation*—a combination of articulation and syllable stress.
3. *Phrasing*—the grouping of words.
4. *Pattern of inflection*—the intonation or contours (melody) of speech.

As listeners, we do not ordinarily analyze which of these factors makes for or detracts from an intelligible message. But any of them, if it deviates too much from what we expect, can make decoding very difficult. This is especially true if the message is long or complicated and we have had little opportunity to "tune in."

The Sounds of Infancy: Early Articulation

Now let us return to the matter of articulation, or the production of the sounds of the child's (really, the adult's) language. Occasionally we discover a beginning speaker, usually a girl, who somehow speaks like an adult with the first words. But most beginning speakers do just what we would expect. They speak like infants, with a very small inventory of sounds. Because infant speakers, presumably, do not have much to say, and because most adults are decently tolerant, infant speech is decodable. That is, babies speak distinctly enough to express their little messages.

If we examine the early messages, the matter about which infants speak, and how these messages sound, we will have a pretty good idea of infant pronunciation. Van Riper (1950) collected the earliest words spoken by American children. In his book *Teaching Your Child to Talk,* he listed the most common words and their pronunciations. The list includes the following:[1]

mama	*mother*
dada	*father*

---

[1] My own recent informal survey indicates that with very few exceptions, Van Riper's (1950) early word list still stands. I would add *ga* (*gaga*) for *doggy.*

bah or *ba-ba*	*bye-bye, ball,* or *baby*
kaaka	*coke* or *crackers*
titta	*tick-tock* or *sister*
puh-puh	*puppy, papa,* or *pipe*
ha	*hat* or *here*
pitty	*pretty*
dih	produced nasally, for *drink*
wah or *wa-wa*	*water* or *bow-wow*
pee or *peek*	*peekaboo*
nanna	*nurse* or some substitute for mother
nuh-nuh	*no*

From this basic vocabulary we can see that a child uses about 15 sounds in his or her first utterances. Ultimately—say, by the age of 7—the child will learn to produce 40 to 44 distinctly different sounds as a speaker of English. The actual number depends on the dialect of English that the child hears and uses.

Many children get along with only 10 basic sounds—a single vowel and nine consonants—for 6 months to a year after they say their first words. By 4 years of age, most of the sounds of the language are under good control. English-speaking children may continue to have some difficulty with the *s, l, r,* and *th* sounds. By 7 or 8, even these difficulties are likely to have been overcome, and children articulate (pronounce their words) much as adults do. Some children, more likely girls than boys, reach this adult-like proficiency by the time they are 5 years old.

A few children, mostly those who have impaired hearing and some who for other reasons are delayed in their speech development, seem to have difficulty with grammar. These children may not say the final *s, t,* and *d* sounds because they don't understand how to form plural words, or words in the past tense, or how to indicate possession.

Occasionally we observe regressions. Even normal children sometimes slip backward in their speech development. It is as if the child recalls that he or she still has the right to speak like a child, to lisp his *s* and *z* sounds, and to substitute a *w* for an *l* or an *r*. These substitutions are called "infantilisms." They may indeed indicate that, for the moment at least, the child wishes to be a baby again, or even that the burdens of childhood are too great. Ordinarily, these infantilisms are but a passing phase in social development. I don't recommend correcting them until the child is at least 6 or

7 years old. Even then, it may be better to deal with the cause—the reason for the child's need to be infantile—than to treat the symptom.

The Sounds of Growing Up

As indicated earlier, most children can "control" most vowels by age 3 or 4 years, but there is considerable variation from child to child. The most important thing to look for is continued progress, whatever the age.

Tongue Trippers

English speech has many combinations or blends of sounds, such as *dr* in *drink, bl* in *blue, st* and *sk* as in *steak* and *skip.* There are also triple-sound blends such as *sks* and *str* as in *asks* and *street.* Even at age 7 years, these blends may not be produced proficiently, although the individual sounds of the blends are under control. Typically, younger children omit one of the sounds or substitute another that is, for them, easier to produce. *Drink* may at first be produced as *dih* and later as *dink* or *dwink* before the child gives it a "grown-up" pronunciation. In the same way, *please* may begin as *pee* and then become *pease* before it becomes a word of four sounds and the *l* is included in its proper place.

Many children, in their early efforts at articulation (pronunciation), reverse the order of sounds. *Ask* may be pronounced as *aks.* A favorite pronunciation is *pasghetti* for *spaghetti.* Some of these "cute" sound-order reversals become family words. But there is a danger involved: The child may be embarrassed when using these words outside the family, as he or she may be misunderstood, or laughed at even when understood.

Common Articulation "Errors"

Most of the pronunciation "errors" that children have follow a certain pattern. Here are a few guidelines that may help parents decode their children's messages:

- Sounds such as *k* and *t* are often interchangeable; so are *d, b,* and *p*; and either *t* or *k* and *d* and *g.* In a child's early speech attempts, one of these sounds may be used for any of the others. Thus, *candy* may be *pandy* or *tandy*.

- A sound used in one part of a word may be used again in another part of the word. So, *dolly* may become *doddy, kitty* may become *titty* or *kicky*, and *Fido* may become *dodo* or *fofo*.

- In general, sounds mastered at an early age are sometimes substituted for sounds mastered later. Table 7.1 may serve as a guide.

- Children perceive certain common combinations of words in a different way than adults do. They perceive them as they are in fact pronounced! So an *apple* may be heard as a *napple*. An early pronunciation may be *nappuh* before it becomes *napple*. Subsequently, the *n* is dropped and the *apple* emerges as the fruit of the articulatory labor.

What should parents do about such "errors"? My answer is, given enough examples of the adult form of any given word, the child will eventually use the adult form. Usually before the child begins to use the adult form, he or she will reject the infantile pronunciation (mispronunciation), showing that he or she is about through with baby talk. Just as the child manages to learn not to say *napple* unless saying *an apple,* he or she will also get the right order of the syllables of *spaghetti* and later of *elephant* and *hippopotamus.*

Children straighten out their listening before "correcting" their pronunciations. Thus, even after the child knows whether the adult has produced the syllables of the word in correct order, the child may still ask mother for *pasghetti.* However, the food may then be refused, or at least the pronunciation for it, if you, too, say *pasghetti.* If you then ask the child what is wanted, *pasghetti* may be the answer. But do not despair! Once the child knows that you are wrong or pretending, correct pronunciation will soon follow.

There are some words that defy many adults. The word *ask* is pronounced *aks* by numerous older speakers. We have also heard highly intelligent and well-educated speakers pronounce *larynx* as *lar niks* and *pharynx* as *phar niks.*

By 18 months of age most children have made two important and related discoveries. Though what they hear from grown-ups is physically a stream of syllables punctuated by occasional pauses, sputterings, and bursts of sounds, somehow they discern that (a) a stream of speech has identifiable words, and (b) the words are made up of identifiable sounds. Before they make these important discoveries, adult speech must sound like jargon to them. Jargon is what we often accuse them of perpetrating. Just what is jargon?

Jargon and the Reasons for It

Jargon is a stage that often but not invariably follows the two-word level of language acquisition. Once children make the discovery that they can identify more than one word in a stream of utterances, they often become jargon speakers—that is, they imitate what they hear. Most adult speakers, quite properly, tend to emphasize the first and last "main" words of a sentence. Usually, these are the words we would retain if we reduced a message to an economical telegram. In most sentences they would include the subject (a noun or pronoun) and the predicate (a verb), and/or the object of the verb. A child might recall the phrase, "Johnny, have one of these nice cookies." At the two-word stage he might reduce this to "Johnny cookie." But though Johnny may not recall all the other words he heard, he does recall that there were other sounds. So, usually with appropriate intonation, Johnny-the-jargon-speaker may fill in the places between "Johnny" and "cookie" with a production of unintelligible sounds that represent to him the flow of adult speech.

Not all children indulge in jargon, at least not to adults. Some speak jargon to their pets. Others speak jargon to themselves before falling asleep. Probably all jargon speakers reveal to us how we sound to them.

Moreover, jargon for its own sake may be fun! We can get some idea of how we sound to young children if we recall how foreigners sound to us when they speak to one another. They all seem to speak with amazing speed. They articulate faster than we can comfortably hear. When we learn a new language, even a few words of a language new to us, the speakers seem to slow down. Actually, it is our hearing/listening mechanism that has adjusted. Even for grown-ups, speaking jargon may be fun; otherwise we would have no songs that go "koo-koo-ka-choo" or "hey nonny nonny." Many of us— or at least our friends and neighbors—do talk admitted nonsense to pets and to innocent children.

Parents should be aware, however, that not all that sounds like jargon are intended as jargon by the child speaker. The adult must try to tune in and do some pronunciation decoding. The guidelines suggested above should help. One way of testing whether the child is using jargon intentionally is to respond with some jargon of your own. If the child seems pleased, then assume it is intended jargon. If, however, the child becomes disturbed, angered, or frustrated at your inability to understand the message, it is not *intended* to be jargon. Then it is your responsibility as a motivated adult to try some decoding. If you don't succeed at first, try again. If you continue to fail, find a better decoder if one is available. If not, show your regret, and, if you can, change the subject.

Some children reserve jargon for occasions that parallel those in which adults would swear, use nonsense language, or talk intimate love talk. That is, children use jargon to express feeling and emotions for which they have no words. As children grow older, they will emulate adults in their use of emotionally laden language and they, too, will learn to say things that are biologically improbable and genetically incompatible. Children will learn how to emit utterances that both question and assert ancestry and posterity. But until children learn this earthy, largely Anglo-Saxon vocabulary, they have to be content with jargon.

Intelligibility and the Role of the Parent: To Do and Not To Do

The intelligibility of a child's speech increases with age. When children are in their one-word stage, usually up to 18 months of age, about 25% of their words are readily intelligible. In their two-word stage, usually between 18 and 24 months, from 50% to 70% of their utterances are intelligible. By 3 years of age, almost all their utterances can be easily understood. However, understanding the child's speech still calls for some decoding, or sound substitutions, by the listener.

By 4 years of age, there should be very little need for sound-substitution decoding. This does not mean that the child is completely proficient in articulation. It does mean that because the child is speaking with conventional grammar and intonation, *messages as a whole are intelligible.* This is so even though some of the child's speech sounds are still not up to the adult level of competence.

What can parents do to help their children speak distinctly? The answers are simple, and most parents do these things quite naturally:

- Be good models as speakers.

- When speaking directly to a preschool-age child, speak in simpler sentences and more slowly than you would to a grown-up child or another adult.

- If a child is not proficient in sound production, do not reject attempts at speaking. Try to understand.

- Do not imitate the infantilisms that constitute baby talk. Be an adult. That is what the child expects.

So, if the child says "Dada pay wadio," your answer, if you are the "dada," is to say, "Daddy will play the radio," or even, more simply, "Daddy plays radio." If you prefer to be a *dada* then, simply, "Dada plays radio." Then be sure to suit the action to the word. When the radio is on, you might then observe, "Radio is playing," or "Radio playing." It won't hurt to exaggerate the *r* sound, but don't make it sound like the growl of an angry dog. A "purr" would be better.

Except by example, parents should not correct their children's speech. Comparatively few children have "defective" articulation as they mature. With good models, nearly all children who are born with the usual sound-producing and hearing equipment learn to articulate proficiently. Almost all so-called errors correct themselves by the age of 7 or 8 years. If a particular child does not become articulate by then, despite good models, then professional help is indicated.

A final caution to parents: Some children have several kinds of difficulty in speaking. They may have trouble in organizing their language, in finding appropriate words, and in using conventional grammar, as well as in articulating. If your child is like this, *do not correct his or her articulation.* This kind of child, even more than others, would be held back by being corrected. Excessive self-consciousness about speaking may produce an insecure, hesitant, halting speaker. Pronunciation may improve a little, but possibly at the expense of overall fluency. At worst, the child may sound like a stutterer.

Chapter 8

Is My Child a Clutterer?

A mother brought her Jesse to me with a perplexing problem about his speech. She said, "Jesse doesn't seem to know what he wants to say, but he is hell bent on saying it." I was impressed by the insight of her terse description of her child's speech and asked her to expand. Jesse's mother not only described the child's speech but also had a tape recording to support her description. She asked, "Is this a form of stuttering?"

At 4 years old, Jesse sounded as if he were trying to talk with a mouthful of hot potato in his mouth. His words were "too hot to handle." Some of the words, mostly the short words, were repeated. Longer words were fractured, and often the order of sounds was transposed so that *water* became *tawa* with the *r* omitted. At best, articulation was approximate. The sounds and the words did not flow and stop places appeared to be random. The hard-to-identify words seemed to come in sputters and bursts. Often even what might have become phrases were left dangling, as if the utterance, however momentary in production, seemed to be out of his control. However, there was little or no awareness of his production. If Jesse were an adolescent or adult, we might conclude that he had a benign indifference about his speech. As I listened, I concluded that Jesse's language production was *repetitious, fragmented, and much too rapid for his ability to articulate.* As a consequence, unless one knew Jesse well, and knew the situation that evoked the utterance, his speech was not intelligible. Another aspect of his lack of intelligibility was his poorly organized phrases and sentences.

In their normal development, all children have periods of hesitant, repetitious speech. All children—at least almost all, let us say, to allow for rare exceptions—also play with sounds and seem to babble for the enjoyment of sound making. Such "speech" is likely to be quite fluent and there is evident enjoyment rather than benign indifference to the speech flow. In contrast, the speech of the clutterer suggests a "tangled tongue" gone out of control. In a broad sense, we might consider cluttering a hyperfluency problem.

To return to the mother's question, "Is this a form of stuttering?" My answer is that there is a superficial common component relative to repetitions. But the repetitions of the child who is stuttering are an effort to deal with a block in fluency, whereas those of the child who is a clutterer are, if anything, overfluent and produced without anxiety. However, in the families of children who have cluttered speech, there may also be stutterers. This may be in related families rather than in their own. There are reported instances that some children who began as clutterers became stutterers. We will address this question later in the chapter after we consider the family background.

Much of how our Jesse speaks also characterizes the casual, conversational speech of adolescents and adults. However, few adolescents and adults provide so few cues in their phrasing and incomplete *but not fragmented* phrases and sentences to make guessing at their *start-out* intended meaning beyond us. Those who do are, like Jesse, clutterers. We may feel about them that they have only a vague idea of what they want to communicate, but are compelled to give it a try.

The Clutterer's Family: A Profile

Our Jesse has a background history fairly typical of children who have cluttered speech. He began to speak at 26 months. He walked at 18 months, but fell more often than most children his age. He bumps into whatever is available for bumping. His mother insists that he goes out of his way to find "bumpable" objects. Almost everything seems to be in his way. At age 4, he was unable to ride a tricycle, much less a bicycle. He can throw a ball, but has not established a preferred hand. At present, he is equally ambi-nondextrous. He can scribble with either hand! Essentially, Jesse is an awkward child. But he has an urge to do things with blocks and crayons and his toys. When Jesse moves, he seems to move "all at once and all of a sudden." His movements seem to be impulsive rather than considered and controlled toward an identifiable objective.

How did our Jesse and other "Jesses" get this way? In almost all instances, they come by it genetically, with a family history, especially on the father's side. The cluttering appears not only in speech, but also later in reading and writing. Even after a preferred handedness is established, writing is likely to be as illegible as speech is unintelligible. Words are often omitted and spelling is poor with many letter transpositions. From early childhood to adolescence and into adulthood we have the impression of their being loosely and tentatively assembled persons, awkward and imprecise whenever physical skills are involved. But—and this is an important *but*—they do not lack in intelligence even though they may have school-identified learning disabilities.

Cluttering and Stuttering Compared

On a superficial level, cluttering resembles stuttering in that both are disorders of fluency. In fact, a small number of children who began their speech history as clutterers do become stutterers, but most do not. The reverse seldom if ever occurs. Children who are clutterers are likely to continue their "tangled tongue" productions well into adolescence and into adult years. Most do improve with therapy, but when they are excited, they tend to regress. But when calm is restored, their speech also calms (slows) down and articulation becomes intelligible.

In my practice, I have had adult clients who were clutterers—to be sure in varying degrees relative to situations—who came to me for "refresher" help. However, in contrast to stutterers, they did not develop any anxiety about talking. Neither did they have any "bogy" words or phrases. Most seem to be ready to talk, and talk, and talk.

Is cluttering a "cousin" to stuttering? The answer is "yes" insofar as both are fluency problems. "Yes" also because both stutterers and clutterers seem to have relatives who either are or were stutterers or clutterers. However, learning problems occur considerably less often in children with a history of stuttering.

In the next chapter we will go into more detail to answer the question, "Is my child really stuttering?" For the present, both cluttering and stuttering are subject to improvement, and in many instances, considerable improvement. Table 8.1 summarizes the similarities and differences between clutterers and stutterers.

Table 8.1

Similarities and Differences Between Clutterers and Stutterers

	Clutterers	*Stutterers*
Family history	May be present especially on the male side.	May be present, much more often in males than females.
Onset of speech	Often delayed.	May occasionally be delayed, but not as often or as long as for clutterers.
Likelihood of awareness	Usually unaware; no evidence of anxiety.	Often aware to level of anxiety.
Feeling about own speech	"Benignly indifferent."	Fearful, anxious.
Likely result of		
(a) speaking after instruction to be careful or	Improvement.	Increase of stuttering symptoms.
(b) interruption and reminder to slow down	Improvement.	Worsens; anxious, tense, blocked speech.
Speaking with awareness of importance of situation	Usually improve.	Usually worsen.
Speaking when relaxed, at ease	Worsen.	Improve.
Reading new material aloud	Better at outset.	Worse; improves with rereadings.
Reading familiar material aloud	Worsen.	Improve.

How To Help the Child
Whose Speech Is Cluttered

What can we do for our Jesses and our Janies to modify if not overcome their cluttered speech? More than most children, they need good speech models with *patience!* They need adults who speak slowly, who articulate clearly. They need adults who can speak in a manner that permits the listener to have a distinct impression that what was being said was the result of organized thinking. There should be no doubt as to when a sentence is begun or when it ends. If possible, the sentences should be short and the phrasing apparent. If necessary, the adult should pretend to be an actor who knows his or her lines and speaks them so that they do not sound memorized.

Children who are clutterers invariably speak better when they speak slowly. Whenever your clutterer does speak slowly, respond as promptly as you can with some indication of approval, but don't make too big a deal about it. Engage the child in conversation and, of course, speak slowly and clearly yourself. If the family is about to go out to dinner and Jesse asks, "Where we goin?" your answer might be, "We're going to your favorite restaurant. What do you think you will have?" You may continue the conversation by asking about a waiter that Jesse or Janie likes, or what you may do after dinner. Short interchanges are much better than long productions.

The adult or older sibling needs to be motivated to be a model who also has the responsibility of indicating when the child begins to speed up even after a good start. I suggest that the parents or other caregiver enter into an agreement that they have a signal that means "SLOW DOWN, I can't listen that fast." One family used touching the right ear as a signal; another used a gentle "touch the chin." Because cluttering is a family affair, the "slow down" signal should be one chosen by members of the family, *including the child for whom the signal is intended.*

Reading aloud to the child by a proficient reader is helpful. Reading might begin with picture books without any printed words. The book page should not have any more than two or three pictures with adequate space between them so as not to suggest crowding or clutter. The reader should say something brief and appropriate about each picture. Conversation should be limited to the selected picture. For example, the picture may show a bird in flight. The reader says, "The birdie is flying," and then asks, "Jesse, point to the birdie that is flying" or "What is the birdie doing?" This conversation may go on to observations about the color or colors of the bird, the bird's nest if it is shown in the picture, and other aspects of the bird. But do not push any conversation beyond a point of interest.

If the child's words are intelligible and generally as "correct" as those of a noncluttering child of a comparable age, do not push for proficiency characteristic of an older age. *Intelligible* means that the message is intelligible and not that articulation is of "normal" quality for children older than age 8. You should certainly accept such syllable switches as *pasqhetti* for *spaghetti,* a pronunciation "error" of high frequency with 3- to 5-year-old children. In time, looks of approval may take the place of immediate "M & M" types of rewards. However, a material reward at the end of a session seldom spoils the day.

Encourage the child to build up a useful store of words and phrases initially related to the reading and conversation about the pictures. You may also build up a store of picture books so that the youngster may choose one that is to his or her liking at the "let's read" session. You may also play the game of Now It's My Choice. This tactic will prevent a limitation of vocabulary based on one or two books. Turn taking has its own social value. Later, read simple stories with a slow but undistorted pronunciation. Provide the child with shared things and activities that you can talk about.

If the child is of school age and shows evidence of cluttered speech, professional assistance is indicated. Many schools have speech therapists who can provide such help. It is important that the therapist does not view stuttering and cluttering as the same problem. *Speech therapy should be directed to helping the child organize his or her thinking into words before saying them aloud.* In time, we hope, he or she may learn to think with the speech flow without a silent rehearsal. But, for the present, the child needs help to make simple statements and ask simple questions that are as intelligible as we have a right to expect of a child of his or her age. We might even settle for a level of proficiency of a child as much as a full year younger. When the child matures enough to sound as if some thinking generally precedes talking, he or she will earn an enviable reputation as a thoughtful speaker.

Following are a few final questions for the parents or other caregivers of a child who is a clutterer:

- Is your household physically uncluttered?

- Is your household one that does not suggest any need to hurry?

• Do you maintain eye contact and look as if you are patiently listening while your child takes time to decide what he or she wishes to say and how to say it?

If you answer "yes" to all of the questions and if your own spoken communications to your child are well-organized statements or questions, then you are doing what you should do to be of help to your Jesse or Janie to overcome cluttering. Your "yes" also implies that the atmosphere and tempo of your home are as free as you can make them to avoid haste and stress. Realistically, I am not suggesting that you become angels, but rather to do what you can to establish an atmosphere of care and calm. Realistically, also, as parents or key caregivers, you are responsible for reducing the likelihood that a child who shows early signs of cluttered speech becomes a confirmed clutterer. It may also be that a calmer home atmosphere would benefit all members of the household.

As a final reminder: The improvement of cluttering should be a family affair. The goals of treatment are not limited to the child. They hold for all members of the family who fit the description of the clutterer and should be shared by those who do not clutter.

In our next chapter, we will consider the stutterer, who also has fluency problems, but of a different nature.

Chapter 9

Is My Child Really Stuttering?

In the last chapter, we discussed fluency disorders and compared cluttering with stuttering. We observed that the child who is cluttering seems to have only a vague idea of what he or she wants to say, but nevertheless is compelled to get started. In contrast, the child who is stuttering experiences anxiety, a fear rather than a compulsion to talk, mixed with the social need to speak.

In this chapter, we will consider the question, "Is my child really stuttering?" This question is entertained at one or more times by concerned parents when their child is in the age range of 2 to 6 years. After age 6, the child who speaks in a manner that might suggest stuttering, or who is more than normally dysfluent, is less likely to stutter. Excitement may still be expressed with dysfluency, but the occasions are less frequent. Normal dysfluency is characterized by repetitions and false starts without anxiety or tension; stuttering is speech with evident anxiety and tension and signs of "struggle behavior." The reduction in dysfluency may be a happy consequence of learning how to organize a sequence of words to make a statement or ask a question before getting the word flow under way. By the age of 10 or 11 years, most children—all but 1% at most—are sufficiently fluent to relieve their parents of the fear that their child might be stuttering. In terms of numbers, about 3 million Americans are stutterers, with varying degrees of severity. At one time in their early childhood, more than 25% of children go through a developmental stage that suggests stuttering, or at least considerable dysfluency. However, as already indicated, no more than 1% of children are identified as stutterers. This percentage decreases to a fraction of 1% in the adult years.

Now we will consider how stuttering begins and how it develops. We will also consider what is essentially a normal manner of childhood speech (dysfluency) that resembles and often is confused with stuttering. We will discuss what parents and other caregivers can do to prevent dysfluency and early stuttering from becoming a chronic problem.

Transient and Chronic Stuttering

All of us can recall occasions when we became dysfluent and may even have sounded like stutterers. These occasions are frequently but not always associated with a need to say something about which we were not secure or certain. Sometimes we need to organize our thoughts and, at the same time, put our thoughts into appropriate words for the listener. If the listener is a person we consider to be important or an authority on the subject, then hesitations and repetitions—the use of "uh, uh," "well, well," "I mean," or an awkward pause may become frequent. "You know," seems to be a favorite filler for many teenagers as well as adults.

However, though an adult may momentarily regard this speech as stuttering, *he or she does not become a stutterer.* A *stutterer* is a speaker who is chronically apprehensive about his or her ability to speak without frequent self-interruptions. These fears are accompanied by self-criticism and anxieties that tend to turn the fears into self-fulfilling prophecies. Young children are not born with apprehensions and self-defeating attitudes, but they are almost all capable of acquiring them.

One of the confounding problems of stuttering is that it doesn't happen all the time. As we have noted, nonstutterers are more fluent in their speech at some times than at others. Factors such as fatigue, stress, pressure for quick responses, and the importance of the listeners or the occasion are likely to make even practiced speakers more hesitant. By and large, the situations that make nonstutterers less fluent are the same ones that make a stutterer more likely to stutter. Any factors that lead to normal hesitations and repetitions are likely to produce considerably more hesitation behavior in young speakers. And they lead to much, much more hesitation in children who are incipient (beginning) stutterers.

It is sometimes hard to distinguish between normal hesitations and repetitions (dysfluencies) and incipient stuttering. Fortunately, several other factors can help us identify the child who is or might be an incipient stutterer, and to distinguish that child from the normally fluent child. We will take them up in the next section. Notice, however, that I have used the term *incipient stutterer* because no child, regardless of the manner of early speech, or of background factors that we shall soon list, needs to become a full-fledged stutterer. Parents should keep in mind that the factors connected with stuttering do not invariably lead to stuttering. Factors in the child's background may match those of stutterers—and the child still may not become a stutterer. If a child has sensitive treatment and care, stuttering can be avoided.

The Truths About Stuttering

Research about children who stutter[1] has been going on for more than half a century in the United States, Great Britain, and other countries of the western world. Here are a few of the facts based on that research:

- There are more boys than girls among stutterers. The ratio is about three to four boys for each girl.

- Stuttering tends to run in families. Families that include a stuttering child are more likely to have relatives who stutter than are families without a stuttering child.

- Families with twins are more likely to include a stutterer than are families in which all children are singletons.

- Stutterers are likely to be somewhat later in beginning to talk than nonstuttering children.

- Stuttering is almost always a problem of early childhood, as it usually begins between 3 and 9 years of age. Only rarely does a child *begin* to stutter in the adolescent years. In fact, onset after age 10 or 11 is rare.

---

[1]In England the term *stammering* is used for *stuttering*. An equivalent term is used in most western nations.

Following are some additional observations about stuttering and stutterers:

- In regard to intelligence, stutterers are on the average as intelligent as nonstutters. On a scale (curve) of intelligence, stutterers are distributed throughout the scale in a "normal" distribution.

- There are no "miracle" cures for stuttering. Nor are there any "hard" explanations for spontaneous improvement.

- Most stutterers improve with speech therapy with qualified speech–language clinicians.

- Stutterers who have improved their fluency are found in all vocations and professions.[2]

Stuttering and the Acquisition and Organization of Language

Now we will apply the information and observations just considered to respond to the question, "Is my child really stuttering?" We will emphasize that even if most of the factors in the "truths" list and other observations may fit a particular child, and even if the child is a "self-interrupter" and may be identified as an incipient stutterer, chronic stuttering is not inevitable.

We will discuss stuttering in more detail and provide guidelines on how to distinguish it from the normal dysfluencies that occur in normal language development. We shall also offer suggestions as to what parents and other caregivers can do to reduce the likelihood that normal dysfluencies will develop into a more chronic problem for both the child and the family.

Many authorities in the nature and development of stuttering have found evidence that among incipient stutterers, speech acquisition is slower than it is among most children who are not so identified. But there are many exceptions. Almost all children who are born under normal conditions have the human-species-specific potential for speech. This was referred to earlier as "the language instinct." I prefer to consider it a normal potential to understand spoken language and in turn, somewhat later, to produce spoken language.

---

[2]Among those stutterers who are superior achievers we have the actor James Earl Jones, author Lewis Carroll (Charles L. Dodgson), novelist and playwright John Updike, statesman and author Winston Churchill, and speech–language problems and childhood speech authority Charles Van Riper.

But some children are more proficient and gifted in this potential than others. Some children are early and relatively fluent speakers. They may begin their speaking careers as early as 8 or 9 months and speak in full "grammatical" sentences as early as 15 to 18 months. By 24 months a gifted few may organize their word sequences (sentences) much in the manner of the adults in their homes.

Children who stutter are likely to be somewhat slow in their speech onset, but not so in comprehension. They may also be somewhat delayed in speech sound (articulation, or pronunciation) development. However, the difference is a matter of weeks rather than months, and many early stutterers are well within the average age range. Comparisons with other same-age children may produce expectations in parents and other caregivers that may translate into anxieties and apprehensions that are, usually unconsciously, shared with the child. Perhaps if parents and other caregivers could learn to accept a limited degree of proficiency in talking—as they well may in other skills—we may reduce the percentage of incipient stuttering to below 1%.

A late-to-start-to-speak child who is hesitant and repetitive may not be at all slow in nonspeaking skills. But he or she is, no matter how intelligent and otherwise skillful, a special child. The child may be special in that for many years, perhaps into adult life, he or she will not be as prompt and proficient at organizing language as most other children of the same age. The child may become a capable and even brilliant writer, like some of my colleagues, and may even become an excellent actor or public speaker, *providing the speech or lines are carefully memorized.* But writing is usually done at one's own rate, and acting and public speaking rarely include unrehearsed repartee. It is in the give-and-take of conversation that stutterers of all ages have their greatest difficulty.

Normal Hesitations Versus Stuttering

Now let's define and briefly describe stuttering and contrast it with normal hesitations and repetitions in childhood speech. A child may be considered to be stuttering if he or she self-interrupts the flow of speech by one or more of the following:

- abrupt hesitations
- frequent repetitions or prolongations of a single sound or a syllable

- maintaining a tense and "sticky"[3] position of tongue, lips, or palate (the articulators)

- any combination of these behaviors in speaking

At the outset, a child may not be aware that the way he or she speaks is in any way unusual. Actually it is just as well that the child lacks this awareness. When all too soon the child becomes aware that he or she is a different kind of speaker, a "different" child, he or she may develop defensive techniques to avoid speaking. Or the child may postpone attempts at speaking even as he or she starts. The child may, in effect, begin an internal struggle that gives subsequent speech the flavor of starting and abrupt stopping, and starting and stopping again.

But not all hesitations and repetitions are stuttering. Not all those who hesitate and repeat their words are necessarily even incipient stutterers. More than 99% of all children, adolescents, and adults engage in some degree of hesitation and repetition as they speak their ongoing thoughts to a human listener. Let us call these hesitations and repetitions "normal hesitation behavior." It is the way almost all of us speak when we are figuring out what to say to share our present and ongoing thinking with a respected listener.

There are a few exceptions among us who somehow are gifted with supernormal fluency, who have "the gift of gab." But most adults, and almost all children, show hesitation (dysfluency) behavior in up to 10% of the sounds and words they produce. Late adolescents and adults may do somewhat better. Some adults repeat and hesitate considerably more than most children, but they still are not stutterers. Most normal hesitations and repetitions are of whole words or phrases, or they are fillers such as "uh, uh," "well, well," "I mean," or "you [yuh] know."

How, then, do we distinguish the stuttering child from the one with normal hesitations and repetitions? One distinction is in the manner of rhythm and flow of speech. Easygoing, "bubbly," and bouncy repetitions—even brief hesitations—do not noticeably interfere with the rhythm and flow of speech. In fact, repetitions may help the child maintain speech flow while figuring out how to share ongoing thinking. Repetitions of this sort usually occur on a full syllable, an entire word if it is a short one, or even on

---

[3]A "sticky" position is one in which contact between the articulators is excessively tight or compressed. To the listener, it seems that the child must exert great effort to break the contact and go on with the utterance.

an entire phrase. So "I, I, I . . ." or "I wanna, I wanna, I wanna . . ." are not at all unusual ways for a child to start a sentence. "S, s, s, see" or "br, br, br, brother" is more indicative of stuttering. In general, we can say that syllable repetition or any *broken word* repetition is in the direction of stuttering, whereas whole-word or short-phrase repetition is well within normal speech. However, either kind of repetition is suggestive of stuttering if it is accompanied by "sticky" positions or obvious tension of the articulators.

Prolongations—stretching out a speech sound—may also be suggestive of stuttering, especially if the prolongation is excessive and frequent, and it suggests tension. Again, almost all of us stretch a stretchable sound such as *m, n, s,* or *sh* occasionally. If, however, while trying to make up our minds about what to say, we say, "I'll see you s, s, s Sunday" or, "I'll s, s, s, ssssee you Sssunday," this is unusual and in the direction of the "abnormal." In general, the longer and more frequent the prolongation, the more the speech is in the direction of stuttering rather than normal hesitations. If the prolongations have the appearance and "flavor" of tense or forced articulation, the likelihood is greater that we are dealing with incipient stuttering.

At this point it is important to emphasize that I have known children between the ages of 2 and 4 and older who spoke for brief periods of time in a manner suggestive of stuttering *but who nevertheless did not become chronic stutterers!*

Though not numerous, there are preschool-age children whose speech is marked by two or more stuttering behaviors in periods lasting several weeks. In between these episodes their speech is normally fluent. Then, "mysteriously," speech becomes normally fluent and is so maintained. For the parents, these are times of transient recurrent anxiety!

What Can Parents and Other Caregivers Do?

Now, what can you as parents do about and for your 3- to 6-year-old child who may be an incipient stutterer? I assume that either by the manner of speaking, or by the child's "profile" and family history, you feel that he or she is indeed prone to stuttering. You are reasonably certain the child isn't demonstrating just the normal speech hesitations. He or she is not only hesitant and a self-interrupter, but is also a word fragmenter rather than a "bubbly" whole-word or phrase repeater. The child is more likely to say "muh,

muh, muh Monday, I, I, I'm gu, gu, gu, going to school" rather than "Monday, Monday I'm, I'm going, going to school." Occasionally he or she seems to prolong and with considerable force emit a sound like "mmmmmmm Monday." Moreover, your young child has a cousin whose family lives in a different part of the country, with whom your family has had no face-to-face contact, who is age 10 and a stutterer. This is evidence that stuttering may run in the family on a hereditary rather than a contact basis.

Perhaps the first thing you as parents can and must do is to get rid of the idea that your child—even if excessively hesitant and repetitive—will inevitably become a stutterer. A predisposition to stuttering and even indications of incipient stuttering do not mean that the child is sure to be a stutterer! If, however, the parents, an older brother or sister, or some other key member of the family group does anything to make the incipient stuttering child aware or anxious about speech, true and chronic stuttering may be the consequence. As a formula of probability, stuttering is the sum of excessive hesitation behavior, plus awareness, plus anxiety. In contrast, hesitation behavior without awareness and/or anxiety is likely to remain within the limits of normal dysfluency. So parents must do all they can to ensure that the child's speech, no matter how dysfluent, is accepted and acceptable.

You don't look at the child anxiously, showing your fear that the words may not come out free of hesitations or repetitions. You remember that nearly all adults occasionally show some evidence of hesitation behavior. If you do not remember or do not believe this, tune in on a radio or TV honest-to-goodness spontaneous interview, and note the amount of normal dysfluency by presumably normal or superior speakers. And you make sure that everyone else—aunt, uncle, grandparent, teacher, or respected friend or neighbor—also helps to keep Keysha from becoming self-conscious about her speech. No one should be contemptuous of the gift of speech. Just be relaxed and grateful for the wonderful things that come out.

Remember that Keysha, who has just come lately to speaking, has even more right to her dysfluencies than the professional announcer, or any of Keysha's relatives who have been talking for many years more than she has. Keysha, or Jesse, for that matter, did not learn to walk without stumbling and falling. But very few Jesses and Keyshas, even those who are a bit on the awkward side, become chronic stumblers.

So, you should have an attitude of benign tolerance. Your attitude is one of accepting what the child can do as a speaker. Really, you have no choice.

Not to accept is not only unrealistic but also likely to produce the very behavior—stuttering—that you by all means want to prevent.

Here are some other suggestions, if you need them, for appropriate behavior if you suspect that your young speaker may be an incipient stutterer. First we will present the "Do Not's" and then some positive, "Do" directives for parents of the incipient stutterer.

Do Not's

• Do not use the word *stuttering* or *stammering* or any equivalent word about your child's speech. If the child does hear such a word, he or she will want to know what it means—and *somehow* will figure out, no matter what you say, that it is not good to be a stutterer.

• Do not tell your child to slow down, to stop and think before speaking, or to "start over again and do it right this time." Nor should you say or do *anything* that will make your child feel or suspect that there is anything wrong with how he or she talks. Speaking a bit more slowly yourself provides a model for the child.

• Do not look at your child anxiously, afraid that the word flow may not meet your hopes for fluency. Neither should you sigh in relief when the child somehow does manage to speak without the usual hesitations.

• Do not ask the child to speak if he or she prefers to engage in some other activity. If you make a mental note, or a written one, about situations that are associated with an increase in hesitation behavior, you can avoid asking or expecting your child to speak in such situations.

• Do not discourage the child from speaking on any occasion when the child wishes to talk. If you can, however, "control" the overall environment so that the child will not feel a need to talk in the situations where, as you have noted, he or she is likely to be excessively hesitant or repetitious.

Do's

• Establish as tranquil a home environment as you can achieve without suppressing other members of the family. Try to avoid or reduce the need for speaking in situations that have heightened excitement or produce frustration (as in some games). Children need to learn to live with and accept occasional frustration. But they do not need to talk during or immediately after experiencing it.

• Listen to your child with full attention and patience. When Luis is talking to you, attend to him at least as much as you would like him to attend to you when you are the speaker.

• Speak to your child in a calm, unhurried manner. However, do not slow down so much as to be "dragging out your words" or with an absence of normal rhythm. Occasionally, your speech should include an easy, bouncy repetition, if only to demonstrate that anyone, even a parent, sometimes indulges in hesitation behavior.

• Keep your child in the best possible physical condition. Illnesses are likely to bring on an increase in hesitation behavior. Expect this and accept it if it happens.

• Expect that your child, like many adults, may have a greater urge to speak than to say anything in particular. Maria may start to say something when she does not have the thought, the words, or the sophisticated devices to complete what she seemed to want to say.[4]

• If your child starts something he or she cannot finish, smile pleasantly and take the child off the hook. One way is to ask an easy question or make an observation to which the child can readily respond. The question or observation should have some relation to the situation the child is talking about. This, however, may require a bit of creative thinking. Your question or observation may refer to an earlier part of the conversation. So, if the conversation with your Maria included talk about a game, or a child with whom she was playing, you might refer again to this event or child.

• If your child appears to be groping for a word, or for a "turn of phrase" to complete a statement, wait a decent time for the word or phrase to come. If it does not, calmly and casually provide the word or phrase. If at all possible, do so by using the word or phrase in a statement or question of your own. This technique has the added benefit of providing a complete-sentence grammatical model that your child can imitate. With practice, the child can even make it part of habitual speech behavior. But remember that children (and adults, too, for that matter) are likely to be most dysfluent when learning and trying out new words or longer, more complex constructions.

---

[4]I have had conversations with adults who, in the middle of a sentence, stopped short, and with a sheepish look, asked, "What were we talking about?"

• Although you should casually provide a word or phrase when your child needs it, don't be in a hurry to intrude and obviously complete your child's thoughts. Give the child a chance and look relaxed while waiting.

• Do all you can to make speaking pleasurable. Engage in "party talk," but talk as an adult. Don't talk down to the child. Tell short, amusing anecdotes and play riddles, especially ones the child can guess correctly. Read to your child, especially at times when you have noted that your child is likely to speak with increased hesitation behavior. Your child will learn that there is pleasure in listening as well as talking.

• If your child asks whether there is anything wrong with the way he or she speaks, or demands to know, "Why can't I speak right?" assure the child that he or she is speaking "right." If the child insists that "sometimes my words don't want to come out," explain that you know and that this happens to you, too. It happens to everyone. Do not go into long explanations, however, that reveal your own anxiety. Most children can easily tell when their parents are worried about something.

• If you need help in understanding or following these directives, consult a competent speech or language clinician in your community. Be sure that the person you consult is qualified and competent. If you are in doubt, call or write to your state hearing and speech association or to the American Speech-Language-Hearing Association (ASHA). The address is 1081 Rockville Pike, Rockville, MD 20852-3279; (301) 897-5700. In Canada, the Canadian Speech and Hearing Association and regional associations can supply names and locations of qualified speech and language clinicians.

The School-Age Child Who Is a "Confirmed" Stutterer

What can we do for the child who, by school age, has become a "confirmed" stutterer? That is, for the child who has come to believe and show by anxieties and anticipations that he or she expects to repeat, hesitate, block, and in general be excessively dysfluent and tense about speaking? Few children become "confirmed" as stutterers before they are of school age. However, I have known 3- and 4-year-olds who, at least by their manner and anxieties, spoke as if they expected to stutter, and so they did. But as already indicated, they were not necessarily destined to continue.

First, I must emphasize that the treatment of the young (school-age) stutterer requires professional attention and not the advice of neighbors, relatives, or friends, however well intentioned they may be. Second, the treatment of young confirmed stutterers should involve all of the grown-up members of the family as well as the child. Parent counseling is a must.

When I counsel parents of stutterers, I have two objectives in mind: (a) to provide information about stuttering and children who stutter and (b) to provide opportunities for relieving parents of their feelings of guilt, anxiety, and hostility—both self-directed and child-directed. Parents no less than children need and deserve time and opportunity to express their feelings, their fears, and their hopes. These burdens should be addressed and shared with an understanding professional person who knows how to listen, remain objective, and respond according to need.

Here are some of the things I try to share with parents:

- Even a "confirmed" stutterer does not necessarily become a chronic stutterer.

- Stuttering is often an "on again" and, fortunately, "off again" phenomenon. If the parents can keep a diary of the situations that turn stuttering on, they may help to keep it turned off.

- Children who stutter are likely to increase their stuttering under any form of stress. This includes the stress brought about by awareness of a need to communicate, to deliver a particular message. Communication cannot, of course, be avoided, but the stuttering child should not be pressured or hurried to deliver the intended message.

- Conflict between stuttering child and parent, or older sister and brother, is conducive to stuttering. It is hardly surprising that such conflicts may be replays of conflicts the parents had with siblings or their own parents.

- Permissive attitudes are likely to reduce stuttering. Rigid, perfectionist ones are conducive to stuttering.

- Almost all children who stutter are able to speak easily and fluently when they pretend to be someone else, when they "act." This is especially so when the child can memorize words and play out a role.

- Children who stutter usually have no difficulty in speaking in chorus (two makes a sufficient chorus), singing, or reciting from memory.

- Children who are confirmed in their stuttering should be encouraged to speak in situations in which they can be relatively fluent. In this way, they may learn that there are situations about which they don't need to be apprehensive. The best way for parents to impress their children about their fluency (no-stuttering) situations is to look approving—a smile will do—after *the child has been fluent.* Do not make a big thing about it. If you do, the wise child may conclude that he must be a mighty bad stutterer at most other times.

Following are a few insightful tips from the Stuttering Foundation of America for talking with the child who stutters:

1. Speak in a slow, relaxed rate in your own conversational speech—but not so slow as to sound unnatural.

2. Listen to what the child is saying. Respond to that, rather than to the stuttering.

3. Give appropriate responses to what your child is saying, such as head nods, smiles, and "uh-huhs."

4. Keep natural eye contact whenever the child is talking.

5. Don't rush the child by interrupting or finishing words for him. Don't let others rush or tease the child.

The address of the Stuttering Foundation of America is PO Box 11749, Memphis, TN 38111-0749; (800) 992-9392.

By way of a review of answers to the question: "Is My Child Really Stuttering?" I will highlight the main points of the discussion. Early dysfluencies occur in up to 10% of the child's utterances. Even more than 10% does not necessarily constitute a first stage of stuttering. However, maintained dysfluencies that are accompanied by awareness, self-consciousness, and evidence of anxiety about speaking and self-interruptions are definitely indications of stuttering. For some children, though, this may be an on-again-off-again happening for several months before the child returns to normal dysfluency.

Dysfluencies in general and the early onset of stuttering are related to several factors for children in the 18- to 24-month age range. (This assumes that the child is not a late starter. Some children, a small minority to be sure, do not begin to speak until well past 2 years. However, these children indicate by their behaviors that their understanding of speech addressed to them is not retarded.)

Now, let us summarize the situations in which stuttering is most likely to occur:

1. The child is responsible for the selection of words to be spoken that are appropriate to the situation and cannot be rehearsed. Unless the child initiates a conversation, he or she cannot rehearse more than the first statement and must accept the responsibility of give-and-take.

2. The telephone is an anxiety producer for most early stutterers and for many without regard to age. Beyond "Hello," there is no way to predict what needs to be said!

3. In general, the amount of dysfluency and manifestations of stuttering varies directly with the meaningfulness (information) of the message.

Following are conditions and situations in which the young child who stutters is likely to be fluent:

1. Content is preorganized and memorized, such as the sequences of the days of the week, months of the year, counting up to what the child has learned, reciting a short memorized poem, or singing a well-memorized song.

2. The child is responding as a member of a group in which there is no identified individual responsibility.

3. The child is speaking to a doll, a stuffed animal, or a live pet who cannot respond except as the child speaks for it.

4. The child is pretending that he or she is another person as one might in role playing.

Early Intervention

Let us assume that because of the frequencies of dysfluency and early indications of stuttering—self-interruptions and word and syllable disruptions—and/or of a family history of stuttering either in the child's own family or of close relatives, therapeutic intervention is recommended. What should the therapy be? There are a variety of positions, theories, and approaches. However, beyond support and assurance that stuttering may be a passing problem, my own emphasis, other than family treatment, is on the need to help the child *organize his or her language.* My model for organization is based on research on normal language acquisition in children ages 2 to 9 years. For the young stutterers with whom we are concerned, we will focus on children ages 2 to 4 years.

My program, presently "in the works," will be called *An Illustrated Language Acquisition Program* (ILAP; Eisenson, 1997). ILAP is based on research conducted at the Institute for Childhood Aphasia at the Stanford University School of Medicine. The program was adapted for children who were late in beginning to talk and slow in their development. I consider this program appropriate for young children who stutter as an approach to helping them to organize their speech in nonthreatening increments.

The original program on which ILAP is based was included in Ingram and Eisenson's (1972) *Aphasia in Children.*

Figures 9.1a through 9.1l show a selection of illustrations from the ILAP, presented in the order of normal language acquisitions. The instruction is, "Tell me about the picture." If the child does not respond, the mother or language clinician tells the child and then asks for a response. The next step is to go to the paired item and go through the same procedure. For a 2-year-old child, the first item might be "Billy drinks." The paired item is "Patty drinks." The resourceful parent or clinician would have several other illustrations of the same construction—a word name and an action related to the name. This might be *doggy, kitty,* or a pet.

We will continue with the 2-year-old as a model, and go on to another construction type. If fluency breaks down, then go back to the construction type that was produced with fluency.

Closing Note

As you are trying to elicit appropriate responses to the illustrated developmental word constructions, I advise flexibility. A child's one- or two-word responses to the constructions may, in fact, be more natural than a longer response. The shorter responses may be what the child is likely to hear at home. For example, an answer to "What's the weather outside?" is more often answered by "It's raining" or just "Raining" than by "It's raining outside."

Another need for flexibility is for pronunciations such as *gonna* for "going to" or *wanna* for "want to." Except for speaking in formal situations, the contracted pronunciations are what we are likely to hear and what most

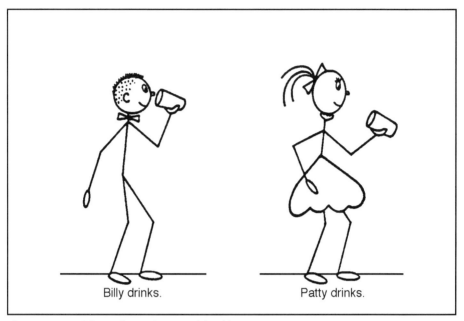

Figure 9.1a.   Noun plus action word (verb).

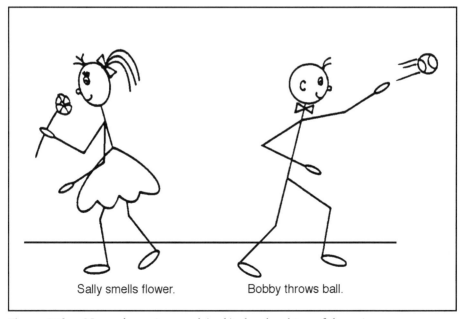

Figure 9.1b.   Noun plus action word (verb) plus the object of the action.

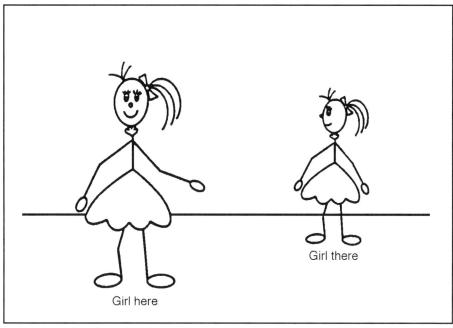

Figure 9.2. Illustration and constructions to establish *here* vs. *there* (noun plus location word).

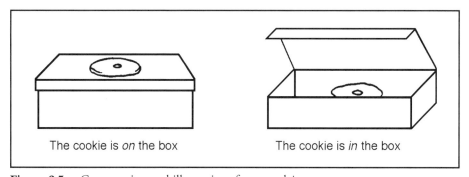

Figure 9.3. Construction and illustrations for *on* and *in*.

of us use. To impose formal pronunciations on a child with fluency problems is unreasonable and likely to be counterproductive. Normal fluency is the objective and so should be the primary consideration for children who are incipient stutterers or are showing signs of early stuttering.

Along the same line as the ILAP is the *Stocker Probe Technique* (Stocker & Goldfarb, 1995). Probes are defined as "grades or level of demand for

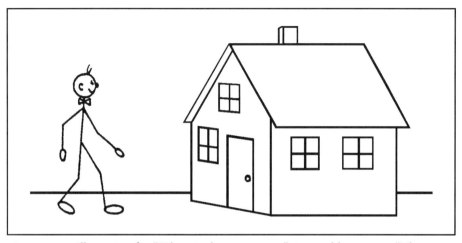

Figure 9.4.   Illustration for "Where is the man going?" Acceptable answers: "The man is going to the house." "To the house."

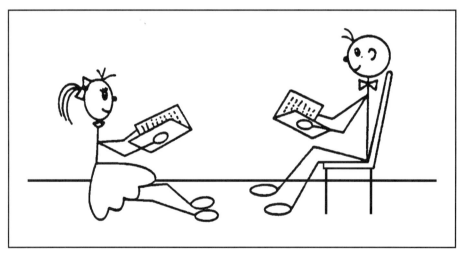

Figure 9.5.   Illustration for "What are the children doing?" Acceptable answers: "They are reading books." "Reading books."

verbal behavior" (p. 7). The probes range from the recognition of and replication of a single word to the need for an increasing number of words in appropriate constructions to making up a story about a common object—ball, lollipop, stamp.

The probes related to the level of demand permit the therapist to determine the level at which to begin to obtain fluency and then how to proceed

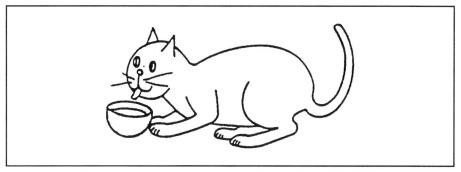

Figure 9.6. Illustration for "What is the kitty doing?" Acceptable answers: "Kitty is drinking the milk." "Drinking milk."

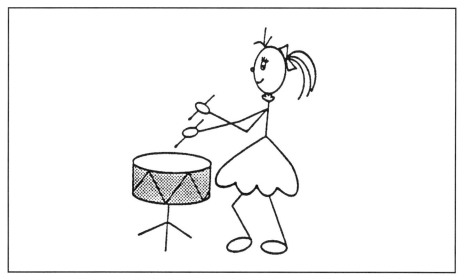

Figure 9.7. Illustration for "What is the girl doing?" Acceptable answers: "The [a] girl is playing the [a] drum." "The girl is beating a drum." "Beating a drum."

from that to higher levels with word constructions to meet the needs of conversational interchange. If fluency breaks down on a given level, the child is "regressed" to a lower level of demand and once again moved forward.

I believe that the *Stocker Probe Technique* shares the assumption underlying the ILAP—that the stutterer needs help in organizing language for purposes of social communicative conversations. This implies a need to be creative in putting words together in statements that are appropriate to the

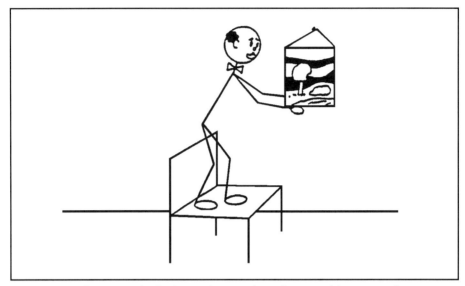

Figure 9.8.   Illustration for "What is the man doing?" Acceptable answers: "Hanging picture on the wall." "Hanging picture."

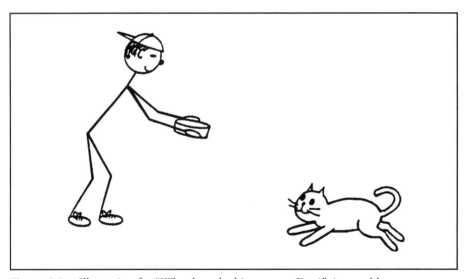

Figure 9.9.   Illustration for "Why does the kitty run to Dan?" Acceptable answers: "The kitty runs to Dan for milk." "For milk." "For water." To encourage a longer response, you might say, "Yes, the kitty runs to Dan for milk [water]"—choose the child's selection.

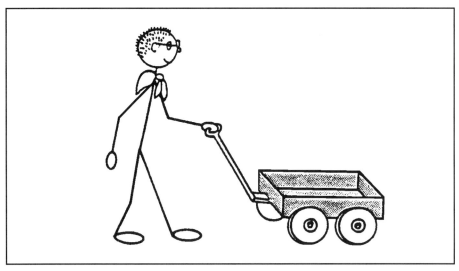

Figure 9.10. Illustration for question sentence with *whose,* as in "Whose wagon is this?" The hoped for response is, "This is Tom's [or other child's name] wagon." But also acceptable: "Tom's." You might try to get a longer response by saying, "Yes, it is Tom's wagon. Can you say that?"

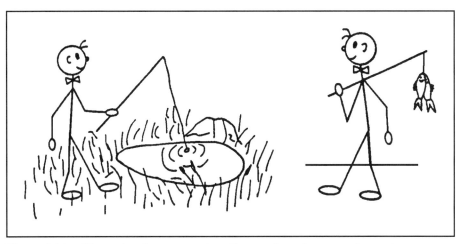

Figure 9.11. Illustration for constructions for questions about ongoing and past actions: such as "What is this boy doing?" "What did this boy do?" Acceptable answers: "The boy *is* fishing." "The boy *was* fishing."

situation. This, of course, is related to the age at which the child began to speak, the models in his or her home, the attention and understanding of the models, and their acceptance of the child's speech. Each child is a law unto him- or herself, and the facility for speech is variable.

The selected readings listed in Appendix 9A could easily be multiplied tenfold. I have chosen a few of the publications that emphasize early childhood dysfluencies and the nature and treatment of young children who stutter.

Appendix 9A
Selected List of Readings on Early Stuttering

Ainsworth, A., & Fraser-Gruss, J. (1975). *If your child stutters: A guide for parents.* Memphis, TN: Speech Foundation of America. (This is one of many publications on stuttering available at low cost.)

Bloodstein, O. (1995). *A handbook on stuttering* (5th ed.). San Diego: Singular Publications. (This is a broad treatment of stuttering by a highly regarded professional teacher and clinician.)

Dell, D. (1979). *Treatment of school age stutters.* Memphis, TN: Speech Foundation of America. (Advice to clinicians and parents, clearly written.)

Conture, E.G. (1982). *Stuttering.* Englewood Cliffs, NJ: Prentice-Hall. (Chapter 3 is devoted to the development and treatment of children who stutter and counseling for parents.)

Eisenson, J. (Ed.). (1975). *Stuttering: A second symposium.* New York: Harper & Row. (Seven clinicians and teachers provide their theories and treatment of stuttering. All include the understanding and treatment of the young stutterer.)

Eisenson J. (1984). *Aphasia and related disorders in children* (2nd ed.). New York: Harper & Row. (Chapter 2 is on normal language development. Chapter 9 has a program for developing language that is applicable to young children who need help in organizing their language beyond the one- to two-word stage.)

Eisenson, J., & Ogilivie, M. (1977). *Communication Disorders in Children* (5th ed.). New York: Macmillan. (Chapter 13 is on the development and treatment of the young school-age child who stutters.)

Stocker B., & Goldfarb, R. (1995). *The Stocker probe technique* (3rd ed.). Vera Beach, FL: Speed Bin. (The *Stocker Probe Technique* was developed for the treatment of young children who are severely dysfluent or identified as stutterers.)

Van Riper, C., & Emerick, L. (1984). *Speech correction* (7th ed.). Englewood Cliffs, NJ: Prentice-Hall. (Chapter 8 deals with the origins of stuttering, its nature, development, and treatment.)

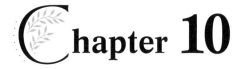

Chapter 10

Is My Child's Brain Different?
Minimal Brain Differences and Attention Problems

"For thousands of years people have tried to understand the brain. The Greeks thought it was like a radiator, to cool the blood. In this century it has been compared to a switchboard, a computer, and a hologram, and no doubt it will be likened to any number of machines yet to be invented. But none of these analogues is adequate, for the brain is unique in the universe, and unlike anything man has ever made."

ROBERT ORNSTEIN AND RICHARD THOMPSON, *THE AMAZING BRAIN*

"The nervous system isn't waiting for birth to flip a switch and get going. . . . The newborn comes equipped with a set of genetically based rules for how learning takes place and is then literally shaped by experience. . . . Associations in early life help choose which synapses live or die. The number of synapses reach adult level by age 2 and continue to increase, far surpassing adult level from ages 4 to 10. The density of synapses then begins to drop, returning typically to adult level by age 16."

"SCIENCE TIMES," *THE NEW YORK TIMES,* AUGUST 29, 1995

Structure and Functions of the Brain

If we could view a living human brain, or for that matter, any mammalian brain, we would see a grayish, indented mass of a substance that resembles soft, mushy clay. The mature brain is about as large as a medium-sized grapefruit and weighs about as much as a medium-sized head of cabbage. With this uncomplimentary comparison, the description ends.

Ornstein and Thompson (1984, p. 21) provided another approach to visualizing the brain: "Form your hands into fists. Each fist is about the size of one of the brain hemispheres, and when both fists are joined at the heel of the hand they describe not only the approximate size and shape of the entire brain, but also the symmetric structure.

The neurons (nerve cells)—about 60 billion, more or less a million or so—are the major constituents of the brain. These cells are "in many ways the most remarkable cells in all biology. Most neurons in the brain are very tiny, some no larger than a few millionths of a meter in diameter, but their numbers are legion. . . . The brain is living—it can grow and change, but a computer can't—and [the brain] is infinitely more complex than present day computers" (Ornstein & Thompson, pp. 21, 83).

Brain Development and Brain Differences

Is my child's brain different? In a strict sense, the answer is: "Of course." We understand that the human brain continues its development for at least 2 years after birth. Although the brain develops according to recognized patterns that include a "wiring system" that specializes in the reception and production of spoken language, no two brain patterns are precisely the same. Experiences, possibly including those as a fetus and certainly in the early years after birth, produce modifications of the "usual" pattern that make no two brains identical.

Most differences in brain patterns may result in only slight variations from "normal" or expected functioning. However, in individual instances, even minor structural (patterning) differences may be associated with appreciable differences in functioning. We will limit our concerns and emphasize the deviations from normal patterning that influence language learning and speech production. These may be a direct consequence of the deviations, incurred congenitally or as a result of injury or disease. For the present, however, let us consider some of the factors and influences that usually produce only slight structural modifications, but that sometimes produce significant differences—not necessarily negative—on functioning.

Any of the following factors may be associated with language acquisition and speech production:

1. dominance of the left or right hemisphere for language

2. age at which a child is exposed to a particular manner of instruction

3. mode of instruction and compatibility with stage and development of cerebral maturation (this correlates with item 2)

4. a combination of any of the above factors.

Any of these factors alone—and more so in combination—may produce psychological influences that generate functional differences that may have a negative effect on speech production. On occasion, when the factors are happily consonant with time and mode of instruction, the consequence may be positive for language acquisition and speech production.

Children go through a series of critical developmental stages. The term *critical* implies that some skills and cognitive development are related to developmental time and stage. Language acquisition begins at birth. Children who for some extraordinary reason are not exposed to speaking persons, or are exposed to persons who speak and relate to them rarely, may not acquire full language proficiency until after age 8 or 9 years, even with great efforts at instruction. More conservatively, such children rarely become as proficient in language as do those who have normal spoken language exposure and relationships with older adults and siblings. The term *critical* also implies an age, almost always before puberty, when the brain is still highly impressionable and not yet rigidly lateralized for hemisphere dominance and related control for language. Thus the best time for a child to learn a second language is in early childhood, and, if possible, no later than 9 years of age.

The term *imprinting* is used by psychologists to refer to the proficient acquisition of a specific skill or a developmental behavior. In the area of language, some psycholinguists consider this to be as early as age 2, but most allow a greater range in time, up to the age of puberty.

The MBD Child and Attention-Deficit Disorders

The child with so-called minimal brain damage (MBD)—more aptly termed minimal brain difference—is probably one whose brain has a difference in structural organization that causes more than a minimal difference in language learning. He or she is also one with *attention deficits* and, more often than not, is hyperactive.

Kinsbourne and Caplan (1979) used the term *cognitive style disorders* instead of *attention disorders* to refer to both overly impulsive and overly compulsive behavior. "Extreme impulsiveness is also sometimes called *hyperactivity* or *underfocused* attention. Extreme compulsiveness may also be called *overfocused attention*" (pp. 3–4). In regard to possible etiology for these attention (cognitive style) differences, Kinsbourne and Caplan noted:

> We know in principle that a lag in cognitive development can derive either from an individual variation in genetic programming or from early damage to an area of the brain destined subsequently to control the behavior in question. In an individual case, we sometimes have enough information to estimate the probability that one of these two general mechanisms is at work, but we have no available procedures that can incriminate either one with certainty. . . . From the therapeutic point of view the distinction is . . . academic, since knowledge of antecedents does not select more effectively from the range of therapeutic options. (pp. 8–9)

The following description of a child illustrates many of the behaviors associated with children who, by neurological evaluation, are confirmed to be brain damaged. In the instances to be presented, there was no neurological confirmation, but the behaviors were all there.

Bobby is a wall climber! He is constantly on the go, disturbing everything he touches, and he touches everything within his reach. And little seems to be beyond his reach. For fleeting moments Bobby pays attention to everything within sight or hearing, but rarely does he pay enough attention to anything. Sometimes, however, he becomes compulsively involved with a toy, a block of wood, or a piece of colored paper, and concentrates on it beyond adult understanding. Bobby appears to have unlimited energy and wears out the adults who care for him. Bobby can't sit still or stand still until he is asleep. Yet, with all the energy he has expended during his long day, Bobby doesn't seem to need much sleep. His parents, unfortunately, do.

What keeps Bobby and the adults who look after him on the run? And why is Bobby likely to be slow in beginning to talk, and later in learning to read and write and in learning what most children readily learn at school? With all the problems Bobby presents, to himself and to his family and teachers, the likelihood is that Bobby does not have mental retardation. He learns some skills remarkably fast, even if they are only the skills of knowing how to get what he wants, to move fast, to get into places he doesn't belong. Somehow we get an intuitive feeling that Bobby is a canny youngster who learns on the fly and knows considerably more than he can tell, or cares to tell.

Other Designations for the Child with MBD

Educators—perhaps more concerned with the problems of learning rather than an often-unsupported medical diagnostic designation—substituted the term *dysfunction* for *damage*. A more recent term, especially for children who do not learn despite presumably adequate intelligence and normal sensory abilities, is *specific learning disability.*

The third edition of the *Diagnostic and Statistical Manual of Mental Disorders* (DSM-III; American Psychiatric Association, 1980) provides several related categories of developmental disorders that include or overlap the preceding designations.[1] These encompass language, speech, and learning disabilities. In broad outline, they are as follows:

- attention deficits
    with hyperactivity
    without hyperactivity
    residual

---

[1]My impression is that the DSM-III categories are overinclusive. On a purely semantic basis, I have a problem with a category that is at once *mixed* and *specific.*

- developmental language disorder
  expressive type
  receptive type

- developmental articulation disorder

- developmental reading disorder

- developmental arithmetic disorder

- mixed specific developmental disorder

- atypical specific developmental disorder

The fourth edition of the *Diagnostic and Statistical Manual* (American Psychiatric Association, 1994) elaborates on the criteria for attention-deficit/hyperactivity disorder. The DSM codes, based on type, are as follows:

- attention-deficit/hyperactivity, combined type

- attention-deficit/hyperactivity disorder, predominantly inattentive type

- attention-deficit/hyperactivity disorder, predominantly hyperactive–impulsive type

- attention-deficit/hyperactivity disorder, not otherwise specified

The DSM-IV emphasizes that the symptoms of hyperactivity should persist for at least 6 months before the diagnosis is made, and that the maladaptive behavior should not be consistent with the developmental level of the child. (For details about the types of attention-deficit disorders, see pp. 83–85 of the DSM-IV.)

Language and the Brain

I offer the following explanation to parents of children with MBD on how the brain functions relative to language and to learning that requires language. My emphasis is on how the brain, and particularly the cerebral cortex, functions in processing (comprehension and production) verbal behavior. Admittedly, it is an elementary explanation—but not a misleading one.

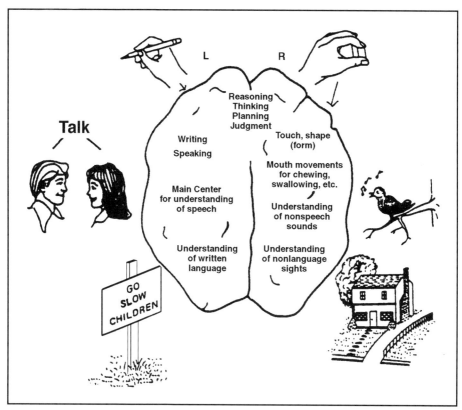

Figure 10.1. Differential functions of the cerebral hemispheres at the level of the cortex with special attention to the language areas (left half) and the nonlanguage areas (right half). *Note.* From *Communicative Disorders in Children* (5th ed.), p. 114, by J. Eisenson and M. Ogilvie, 1983, New York: Macmillan. Copyright 1983 by Macmillan. Reprinted with permission.

The brain, or cerebrum, is divided into two halves (hemispheres) that superficially are more alike in appearance than most identical twins. But there are differences in structure that are related to differences in functions and responsibilities. The hemispheres are different, but, in significant ways, still related, as shown in Figure 10.1. For example, both hemispheres have areas concerned with sound: The left hemisphere, for almost all of us, deals with the sounds of spoken language; the right hemisphere deals with processing nonspeech sounds, such as mechanical noises, music, and even nonspeech human sounds. When we learn the words and music of a song, the left hemisphere learns the words and the right hemisphere learns the melody.

Visual images are received by areas in the back of the brain cortex. The right hemisphere is involved with images that do not require verbal decoding. But if the images are recognized as written words, their interpretation (reading) requires the specialized function of the left hemisphere.

As another example, the movements for chewing and swallowing are controlled by an area toward the front of the right side of the brain cortex. Movements for speaking, however, are controlled by an area located toward the front of the left side of the brain.

Note that, in all these examples, the left side of the brain is normally the one involved in language functions. This is the case for understanding and producing speech, as well as for learning to read and write. Almost all right-handed adults have this kind of control or dominance for language. Left-handed persons represent an interesting minority. About 50% of all left-handers appear to have language functions, and probably other functions as well, controlled by either or both hemispheres. The other 50% seem to have control or dominance on the left side, about the same as right-handed persons.

The control or dominance for language is established at about the same age that children show clear preference for handedness. Thus, though one is not the cause of the other, hand preference and brain dominance for language develop together. By 3 years old, most children are clearly either left-handed or right-handed. A very small percentage are truly ambidextrous—that is, they can use either hand with almost an equal degree of skill. Another very small percentage are almost equally *unskilled* with both hands. In this small population, we find children who are slow in acquiring speech. We considered some of them in our discussion of cluttering (see Chapter 8).

The brain cortex contains billions of nerve cells, or neurons. Some of these cells are specialized and concentrated in areas or centers for special functions, as already noted and indicated in Figure 10.1. Other cells serve as conductors of impulses from one center to another and from one hemisphere to the other. Thus, we can talk about what we see, imitate the sounds we hear, monitor the sounds we produce, or even reproduce the sounds of the images that are stored in our minds.

The brain cortex makes sense out of sights and sounds. In this respect, it is like a huge computer and switchboard that can deal with what our senses take in. It also enables us to organize the movements needed to produce our own sights and sounds, whether walking, running, speaking, writing, or whatever else a human being is capable of understanding and doing.

The Cerebral Cortex: Attention, Judgment, Reasoning, and Planning

The cortex of the brain is, at least up to now, the crowning achievement in human development. If the crown has any one area that makes it possible for us to behave humanely as well as humanly, it is the area in the front of the brain. The front or forebrain is larger in the human being than in any other primate. This area is responsible for planning, for exercising judgment, for reasoning, and for appreciating the consequences of our behavior.

In the forebrain, we make decisions, such as, "If I do this, the consequence may be. . . ." In the forebrain, we do our planning, including the planning of a sentence to be spoken or written. There also, as we have indicated, we can anticipate what may happen if we say something or write something. The forebrain is the "If I" or "Suppose I" portion of the brain.

What happens if this area is damaged by injury or disease? The results, as known from actual cases, is a disturbance in the planning, judgment, and reasoning abilities.

Suppose—and now we speculate—that the frontal brain area does not develop on schedule. Then we may have an impulsive child who acts without regard to consequences. We may also have a child who is slow in acquiring speech because, as I have indicated, every word to be spoken requires the execution of a plan. For speaking, or for writing, the plans determine what sounds or letters constitute words, and what words are to be selected in a particular order to make a sentence. All this is in keeping with a master plan called *language.* Children with damaged or underdeveloped forebrains have a difficult time doing any of this important planning.

The Child with MBD Who Does Not Talk or Is Slow to Talk

About 30% of all hyperactive children can be diagnosed as having actual brain damage. These children are at the extreme. But moderately hyperactive children are not brain damaged, at least by medical standards. As we suggested earlier, they are probably brain different. What kinds of behavior do these children demonstrate? Most of them show the following:

- They usually are well within the average or above-average range of intelligence. This finding is supported by several psychological studies.

- They have trouble paying attention, especially to the words that people say to them.

- They are often impulsive and frequently difficult to control.

- They may be awkward and slow in developing body skills, including walking, running, hopping, and climbing.

- They are likely to be slow in developing skills such as building with blocks, managing a crayon, or dressing themselves.

- They are very slow in understanding language and in learning to talk. Some who do learn to talk may have difficulty in learning to read and write.

These children with MBD who have difficulty acquiring language represent a very small percentage, really a fraction of a percent, of all children. Some will pay attention quite appropriately to the sounds of pets and to mechanical sounds but seem to ignore speech. This may be explained by our knowledge that nonspeech sounds, including those made by so-called talking birds, are "processed" in the right hemisphere of the brain. Speech, as we have learned, is usually controlled or processed in the left hemisphere. A child may be telling us, by the sounds he or she pays attention to and by those he or she seems to ignore, that his or her left hemisphere has not matured sufficiently to be able to decode human spoken language.

In an extreme case, a child like this may be designated as *aphasic,* or nonspeaking. If the problem of language learning is not severe but just mildly delayed, the child is said to be *dysphasic.*[2] Fortunately, we know considerably more about such children than we did when their mothers were children. Fortunately, also, a considerable amount can be done for them by direct teaching of small and selected units of language. These units have

---

[2] The term *dysphasia* is generally used in Great Britain and Europe for hearing children, presumably within the normal range of intelligence, who are nevertheless significantly impaired in the comprehension and production of language.

been used in programs that parallel the speech development of normal infants and children. One such program is explained and illustrated in *Aphasia and Related Disorders in Children* (Eisenson, 1984).

However, I urge parents not to come to hasty conclusions about whether their child is aphasic or dysphasic. These children and their parents are entitled to professional evaluation and assistance from medical, educational, and language personnel who specialize in child language problems.

Why Some Children with MBD Do Not Talk or Are Slow to Talk

Now let us consider why children who are brain damaged (as diagnosed by a competent physician) behave the way they are likely to. I say "likely" because one of the outstanding characteristics of these children is their changeability. Further, we know that some children with brain damage seldom if ever behave the way that most other children with brain damage typically behave.

Damage to the cortex of the brain often produces extremes in excitability. At one extreme, the child is in a constant state of excitement, responding or attempting to respond to everything within sight, hearing, smell, or touch. At the other extreme, the child may respond to almost nothing; the child stares off into space or is excessively sleepy.

Another effect of damage to the brain cortex may be a compulsion to continue responding to just one thing, one event, to the exclusion of all others. The child's attention may become limited to something the adult considers trivial: a piece of string, a block of wood, or a button on a shirt or dress. Nothing that is important (at least from the adult's point of view) enters the child's awareness.

For a child to acquire language, to learn to speak, the child must be able to pay attention to a speaker long enough to decode what the senses have taken in. If the child's attention span is too brief, if he or she pays attention for just a moment to everything but not long enough to any one thing, the child cannot take much into the mind or store it there. If little or nothing is stored in a mind, there is little or nothing to remember and recall. So, in an extreme case, the child will not be able to learn the language and will not speak.

However, I caution parents that some children who are constantly on the go pay attention to considerably more than we give them credit for.

They seem, literally, to learn on the fly. They do learn language, but seem to be too busy to speak to anyone.

Within the entire population of children with brain difference (not just those that are brain *damaged*) are a fair number who are slow in developing hand preference. They also seem to have trouble dealing with experiences that require them to take things in through more than one sensory avenue at a time. Sights that make sounds, such as a bell, may be disturbing because the child cannot readily make the connection between sight and sound.

We can only speculate that the reason for this is that the nerve cells or fibers that connect the brain centers for sight and sound may not be adequately developed. The timetable for the normal functioning of the specialized brain centers, and that of the conduction fibers, may be delayed compared with that of most children of the same age and potential intelligence. If there is an asynchrony, children with brain difference take in experiences differently, respond to them differently, and learn differently.

Advice for Parents of a Child with MBD

What parents should do for a child with MBD who is hyperactive and distractible is a matter that requires highly expert and specialized advice. By all means, parents should consult a physician and, if possible, a pediatric neurologist. In many instances, children with hyperactivity will benefit from medications that are *prescribed and carefully supervised by a physician.* Highly specialized education should also be considered. Also, parents usually benefit from counseling as soon as the child's basic problem is identified.

If the child with MBD does not understand speech by 18 months at the latest, or understands spoken language but is not speaking by 3 years of age, preschool education with emphasis on language learning is in order. Many schools now have such programs.[3]

This discussion of hyperactivity and its *possible* implications may be anxiety producing for some parents, including those who may have gone for a consultation about a child who has already been labeled hyperactive. Before the label gains the prestige of a diagnosis, several questions need to

---

[3]Public Law 94-142, the Education for All Handicapped Children Act (1975), mandates that school systems provide educational opportunities in the least restrictive environment for every child, regardless of disability. Children with learning disabilities are included under this law.

be asked: When is the child hyperactive? What is your basis for comparison, for deciding that the child is hyperactive? Hyperactive compared with whom? Under what circumstances? Many children, boys more often than girls, become fidgety (hyperactive?) when they are expected to attend to a situation beyond their span of attention. They may, in fact, have obtained all that they want out of the situation. Their fidgeting and restlessness indicate that they are ready for something else. But their parents, and later their teachers, may be working on a different time schedule.[4]

In consultations with parents, I remind them that almost every child is hyperactive (restless) on some occasions. Waiting to go somewhere or to start playing a promised game are typical situations that generate restlessness. Unless the occasions are so frequent as to be beyond generous limits of expectation, there should be no cause for anxious concern. However, occasional and unexpected expressions of excitability should be noted. If such episodes increase in frequency, medical consultation is in order. Chronic hyperactivity may be an indicator of MBD, but it need not be, especially if the child is not deficient in learning.

Parents also become anxiously concerned about a child who, perhaps because the world is too much with him, ceases to pay attention to the situation at hand and becomes compulsively involved with something trivial. This may be an indication that the child needs to "turn off" from environmental demands and "recuperate" from excessive intake. It may be a needed "time-out" period. If, however, such behavior becomes frequent and chronic, then medical consultation is in order.

To sum up, children appropriately diagnosed as MBD require highly specialized professional attention. Experience indicates that most children with MBD benefit from specialized educational programs and some from medical treatment that reduces hyperactivity and enhances attention span and opportunity for learning. Such medical treatment should be supervised by the prescribing physician. I remind parents that there are many causes and many possible treatments for children who are brain different. The diagnosis, and certainly the treatment, should not be made by the parents or by any relative or friends, unless they are professionally trained. Even then, it would be wise to make a referral.

---

[4]Ross (1977, chap. 13) reviewed the literature on studies of presumably hyperactive children. In one study, 49.7% of boys in kindergarten and primary school classes were described by their teachers as "restless and unable to sit still." This percentage would suggest that restlessness is the norm, or very close to it.

No matter what term is used, children who are brain different are not necessarily brain damaged, though about 30% of them may be. But many children who are brain different are "off schedule" in the development of expected behaviors, of which language acquisition is at the outset most prominent. Unfortunately for such children, adult expectations are governed by what most children do, and not by what children who are brain different demonstrate that they can or cannot do. Fortunately, most children who are brain different, including those designated as MBD, catch up. Their cerebral centers develop functional circuitry, and their capacity to deal with events that come to them through all of their senses also catches up. For some children, catching up may occur by 8 or 9 years of age, and for others, by puberty.

Appendix 10A
Selected Readings

Bradley, R. A. (1990). *Attention deficit disorders: A handbook of diagnosis and treatment.* New York: Guilford.

Goldstein, S., & Goldstein, M. (1990). *Managing attention disorders in children.* New York: Wiley.

Kirby, E. A., & Grimley, L. K. (1986). *Understanding and treating attention deficit disorders.* New York: Pergamon.

Psychology Today. (1985, November). (This issue contains several articles written by authorities in their fields on the brain, its structure and functions, with particular attention to language.)

Ross, A. O. (1980). *Psychological disorders in children.* New York: McGraw-Hill. (The author, a psychologist, views attention deficits and hyperactivity as behavior manifestations and educational matters, not necessarily as problems. "Any intervention aimed at reducing hyperactivity must include a systematic plan to replace the hyperactive behavior with goal directed, attentive, and constructive behavior.")

Chapter 11

What Does My Child's Voice Tell Me?

We will begin with a reassuring note. The answer to the question posed by this chapter title is, "A lot." Early sound making and speech are variable. Parents often become anxious about their children's speech, yet chances are that their child's speech is normal, assuming that the child entered the world under normal conditions and made his or her presence known by crying just loud enough and long enough to signal, "All is well and let's get on with it." Without asking for it, the child seems to establish basis for binding and bonding with the mother. (We discussed binding and bonding in Chapter 3.)

Because of this bonding, the caring mother has a unique responsibility for the child's early sound making and the avoidance of voice problems. Doing what comes naturally is really all that is involved. Most voices are essentially normal even though not all of us qualify for the poet Byron's praise, "Like music on the waters is thy sweet voice to me."

In this chapter we explore the many factors that influence a person's speaking voice: its melody or its harshness, its nasal or metallic qualities, its lilt or its mellowness. The quality of a person's voice begins when he or she is still a tiny infant, listening to the voices of others. Later on, a child echoes the voices that he or she hears. But the echo, unless it is the voice of a talented vocal imitator, is and remains the child's own voice.

Early Responses to Voice

Nothing is more distinctive in the behavior of infants than their responses to human voice. Within the first few weeks of life, the baby will respond differently to the voice that purrs and the voice that snarls, to the happy voice and the angry voice. Very early in life, sometimes as early as 3 weeks, the baby may engage in a "dialogue of cooing" with a "cooing" mother. The baby may even learn to wait and take a turn, as becomes a good conversationalist. Angry voices literally "turn babies off." A baby may turn away from the voice or begin to cry. In contrast, the baby is "turned on" and toward the producer of the happy voice, especially if the happy voice is a familiar one. An unexpected voice may produce crying. The sound of the mother's voice may change the crying to cooing, and later, when a child is more "sophisticated," to smiles and laughter.

The baby's early responses to human voice are different from those to any other sounds or noises. We cannot be certain why this is so. It is simply an aspect of what it is to be born a human being. Birds are responsive to other birds' noises, and so singing birds learn to sing. Dogs bark; cats meow. Human beings vocalize and talk. Children who are born with normal equipment are "prewired" to be responsive to human voices. They are also equipped and constructed to make vocal sounds that are expressions of feelings: tender or furious, loving or hateful. They learn to use their voices to cajole or reject, seduce or repel. The voices of human beings can express subtleties beyond the meaning of words. They can even replace words when feelings or meanings cannot be verbalized.

The evolutionist Charles Darwin believed that this very human ability represents an instinct of sympathy. Beginning in infancy and continuing throughout life, voice is the primary way in which human beings show their feelings and emotions. So the child, with an instinct of sympathy, is in special tune with other human voices and uses his or her own voice to express feelings and emotions. This is a also an expression of the language instinct.

Other than crying, how does the normal infant vocalize in response to new noises and new voices? On the basis of my survey of recently published research, following are some of the ways the infant may respond:

- By the end of the first month, the baby cries when exposed to loud noises. The baby may make it a duet when he or she hears another baby crying.

Table 11.1

Early Vocal Responses and Productions Before First Words

Approximate Age	Baby Hears or Sees	Baby Responds
Birth–2 months	Loud noise	Cries.
	Baby cries	Cries.
	Eye contact with adult	Coos, reflexively yawns, gurgles, coughs, sneezes, coos when content. May produce sounds such as "ayruh" when distressed.
	Angry voice	Baby cries and may turn away from voice.
	Nonangry voice	Coos in response.
2–3 months	Sees face or hears familiar voice	Chuckles, laughs.
	Unpleasant voice	Cries.
4–5 months	Social play with adult, tickling	Laughs, as for an older child. "Sings," coos when child is alone and content.
6 months	Speaking person	Variety of vocal responses to indicate feelings. May "exclaim" to show delight. Child responds and imitates differences in vocal melody (intonation) patterns.
7–9 months	Presence of familiar person	Child's vocal contours (melody/intonation) suggest requests, demands. Sophisticated cooing expresses calmness and contentment.
10 months	Adult voice	Child responds by adjusting own pitch level in direction of the voice pitch of the adult, higher when responding to female than to male voice.

Note. Adapted from the following sources: *Infant Speech*, by M. M. Lewis, 1951, New York: Humanities Press; *The Child Who Does Not Talk*, by C. Renfrew and K. Murphy, 1964, London: Heinemann; *Intonation, Perception, and Language*, by P. Lieberman, 1966, Cambridge, MA: MIT Press.

- An adult voice, if it is not an angry voice, will have a soothing (quieting) effect on the baby.

- In the first or second month, the infant responds to a vocalizing adult by smiling. Often the baby will "hold a dialogue" with the adult, "cooing" back to the adult. The baby may start the "cooing" if the adult stops, and so "keep the dialogue going."

If the caregiver or visiting adult does not respond, the cooing may increase in intensity, or may give way to a whimper, or a trial suggestion of a cry until the dialogue is resumed. However, the infant may decide, "I guess I've had enough for now," and fall asleep. But don't count on it.

It is clear that the normal child needs to hear human voices, and responds to human voices in different ways—according to what the voice expresses—very early in life. Favorable conditions, such as hearing human voices often, especially ones with soothing qualities, reinforce the infant's natural tendencies to vocalize. Conditions may also reinforce tendencies to be frightened or to be unhappy, if the baby's experiences are with unhappy or angry voices. These voices, of course, come from unhappy or angry persons.

Table 11.1 summarizes the vocal responses of infants to noise and voice from birth to 10 months.

Motherese and the Melody of Speech

Motherese is what caring mothers "intuitively" say and sing to their babies while they are engaged in necessary caregiving. What they say while they do whatever they need to do changes as the infant becomes the baby and the baby becomes a child. What they "say" may be just words or nonwords set to little tunes that are the melodies (intonation) of speech.[1]

For example, "All gone," says mother when the last spoonful of cereal has gone down the hatch. "Upsy baby," she says when she picks up her baby for burping. Each of these caregiving exclamations is produced with a melody appropriate to the words and the action. Thus, "all gone" is produced as

---

[1]Fathers are not exempt from speaking motherese, but most of them are too self-conscious to be proficient at producing the little tunes that seem to come easily for mothers.

all gone

and "upsy baby" as

upsy baby.

By her words and accompanying speech melody, the mother is in effect teaching her child that there are patterns of speech melody (intonation) that go with a flow of sounds that later will become words. Well before they say their first words, most babies can distinguish upward and downward melody contours. So it is no surprise that their first words are accompanied by the melodies that they have heard grown-ups speak. Students who have studied normal babies find that adult speech melodies are produced in sound play from 1 to 3 months before they say their first words. The speech melodies extend a baby's repertoire beyond the vocal expression of feelings and emotion. In an important sense, the melodies are there, and when the first words are evoked, the words and the melodies are ready for each other.

When the words are produced, we can accept as a truism that there is a very close relationship indeed between the way the children hear words and the way they themselves begin to use them (Harris 1987). This observation is based on Harris's long-term study of children's first words. This brings us back to the opening of the chapter, when we considered the responsibilities that come with child-to-mother bonding. However awesome the responsibility, it can also be delightful.

Following is a motherese interchange between an 18-month-old child who was putting two and three words together to make sentences:

CHILD: (Pointing to a picture of a kitten from one of his favorite books.) "That kitty."

MOTHER: "Yes, that is a kitty."

CHILD: "That is kitty."

MOTHER: "Yes, that is kitty."

The mother decided not to give the child the complete construction: "That is a kitty." She left that for the following week, when the child pointed to the same picture and said: "That is kitty." The mother responded with, "Yes, that is a kitty." The boy then agreed, "That is a kitty." The mother then showed the boy a picture of a dog and then a duck, and for each asked, "What is that?" The child answered with the expanded sentence, "That is a doggy" and "That is a duck." Good motherese; good learning!

Personality and Voice: The Role that Parents Play

Up to this point, we have considered the natural and intuitive way that babies and young children respond to the voices they hear. We have also seen how they express their feelings, their frustrations, their contentment, and even their joy of being alive. In a very real way, babies reveal their budding individuality. We can identify the cranky, colicky baby through excessive crying. The calm, contented baby reveals personality through dovelike cooing. The lively baby earns a reputation through wide-ranging, happy-sounding vocalizing. The demanding baby has a voice that exclaims, commands, and demands loudly and assertively, with falling inflections.

I hesitate to say that "children are born that way," but they do seem to have natural tendencies. However, a voice pattern requires considerable practice and reinforcement before mere tendency becomes entrenched. More often, it seems that the child, because of an inborn capacity to identify and respond to human speakers and their voices, is "shaped" by the voices he or she hears. The chief "shapers" are parents and older brothers and sisters—especially parents. At this point, I encourage parents to ask themselves a number of frank questions. The more objective their answers, the more helpful the results may be, not only for the child, but also for themselves.

First, have you ever heard your own voice as others hear you? Unless you have heard yourself played back on a high-fidelity recording by an equally high-fidelity instrument, your answer should be "no." If it is "no," then have a "candid" tape recording made of your casual speech with an adult and another made when you are talking to your child. Which is the real "you," the personality you wish to project? Is it you talking to another adult? Is it you talking to the child? Can you deny that this is really you on tape? (Some adults first deny and then reluctantly accept the reality of hearing their own voices. The result of hearing ourselves as others hear us may be traumatic. But it can also be highly therapeutic.)

Now, having heard your own voice, what does it tell you? Is it unnecessarily loud? Is it hard, metallic, harsh, or husky? Does it sound as if you are complaining, with whining tones? Or does it sound as if you are making demands when what you really intend is to make a polite request? Do you sound apologetic or self-demeaning when there is no need for such an attitude? Is your voice thin (weak) rather than full? Do you sound as if you are almost out of breath? Is your voice in general—in quality, pitch, force, and intonation—the *you* that you want to express and convey? Most important, is your voice the kind you would want the child you love to imitate?

In my experience, both as a psychologist and as a speech pathologist, I have often had to make parents aware that it is not the child but the mother or father who needed treatment for a voice problem. On numerous occasions I have pointed out to parents that their child must love them a great deal, because the child sounded so much like them. And I proved the point with voice recordings. On most occasions, the way to treat the child was to treat the parents. Sometimes, just by listening to their recorded voices, parents were motivated and able to improve the quality of their voices. Some needed help.

Physical Causes of Voice Problems

There are some voice problems for which parents are not responsible by their example. Children who have frequent colds or allergies that produce nasal congestion have *denasal* voices.[2] Enlarged adenoids produce the same effect. When a cold or any other upper respiratory infection involves the back of the throat (pharynx) or the voice box (larynx), the result is usually a harsh, breathy voice. Vocalization may also be accompanied by considerable pain.

In contrast to the denasal voice is that of a child born with a cleft palate, or with a short soft palate. The voice is then characterized by excessive nasality. We may notice this quality in ourselves if we speak when very tired. Nasality occurs in children as well as adults who are chronically fatigued.

---

[2]Many persons refer to the voice quality associated with "stuffy nose" as *nasal*. This is both illogical and incorrect. When the nasal cavities—the chambers above the roof of the mouth—are clogged because of a cold or an allergy, the voice lacks nasal resonance and so is denasal. We can produce the effects of a denasal voice by pinching the nostrils and saying, "My mother may come to see me." The words may sound more like, "By bother bay cob to see be."

And there are other physical conditions associated with nasality. Parents have an obvious obligation to seek medical advice for any possible physical condition that may account for the problem. If the physician decides that there is no physical or medical problem, then the parent should ask, "Is my child imitating me? Or if I am not the model, is it a playmate or an older member of the family?"

Children who have a history of being *screamers,* who yell rather than talk, may develop thickened vocal bands or little noblike growths (nodules) on their vocal bands. The result is pain when talking and, ultimately, a low-pitched, breathy, hoarse voice. Whether the child's excessively loud voice and its consequences started in some illness or in imitating another person, the parents should seek medical advice and treatment for the child. Not to be overlooked is yelling at games, in the playground, or even in the child's own backyard. (Figure 11.1 shows a drawing of vocal nodules.)

Children who are moderately or severely hard of hearing may speak in a monotonous voice. Children who are lacking in physical vitality, who are chronically tired, are likely to speak with voices that are weak and rather "flat." Again, medical advice is indicated. However, if there is no medical cause, the probability is that the child is imitating a friend or an older admired member of the family.

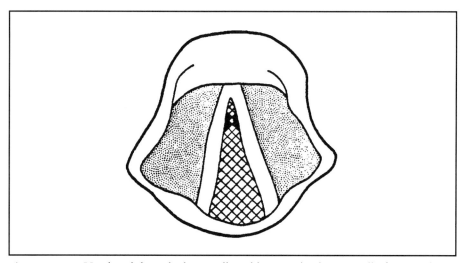

Figure 11.1.   Vocal nodules, which are callous-like growths that typically form in the upper middle third of the vocal bands. Vocal nodules are most often associated with the high-pitched screaming.

If treatment is indicated, it should include the person who is providing the poor example.[3] With children who are younger than school age, the changes in voice will be spontaneous *as long as the model improves.* Children of school age may need direct voice therapy by a professional therapist. We are emphatic in insisting that no child, and for that matter, no adult, should be involved in voice therapy *without a medical evaluation and clearance.* If possible, the evaluation and clearance should be the responsibility of a laryngologist. It is not likely—or advisable—to try to change voice habits until physical problems are first cleared.

The Adolescent Voice: What Parents Can Do

Our emphasis throughout this book has been on the young, preschool child. However, because boys frequently (and girls sometimes) have voice problems when they reach adolescence, we need to consider this aspect of vocal development as well. The basic question is, "Is my adolescent's voice normal?"

Beginning at about 12 or 13 years of age, the voices of boys and girls change markedly in pitch and quality. The changes associated with physical growth and maturity are almost always greater in boys than in girls. In males, the vocal folds (cords) increase about one third in length from early adolescence to adult age. The vocal folds also increase in thickness. Because the range of pitch of the voice becomes lower as the length and thickness of the vocal folds increase, the overall result is that the late male adolescent's voice drops about one octave. In girls, there is a much smaller increase in vocal fold length and thickness. The change in pitch range is therefore not nearly as great.[4] There is, however, a significant change in the quality of the adolescent girl's voice. Normally, the voice is richer and fuller than in childhood. The "ring" of childhood is replaced by the mellowness of maturity.

---

[3]A medical colleague to whom a child was brought for treatment for loud voice took a dramatic-traumatic approach to the problem. He noted that the mother's voice was so loud that it was painful to listen to her. The physician asked the mother whether she had a telephone at home. The mother, surprised, answered, "Of course, why do you ask?" To which the physician replied, "I should think you wouldn't need a telephone, at least not for local calls. All you have to do is open your window and talk away." The mother, we are informed, got the point.

[4]Adult male vocal folds range from 7/8 to 1 1/4 inches in length. Adult female vocal folds range from 1/2 to 5/8 inch. The longer the vocal folds, the lower the pitch.

Girls' voices may change in richness and mellowness, but most boys almost literally obtain new voices. Once they played with voices in the range of the violin; during adolescence they must learn to deal with instruments that have a cello or bass fiddle range.[5]

For a while, boys' voices may seem to be out of control. They may become hoarse and husky, or breathy. They may "break" in pitch and become falsetto. Suddenly and unexpectedly, even to the boy himself, his voice may go from a preadolescent high pitch to a treble to a husky bass. In a very real sense, it is as if a familiar musical instrument has become defective. It is as if someone had placed the reeds of a bass instrument into one intended for a considerably higher pitch range, such as a French horn, without informing the musician of the change. The instrument is literally out of tune. But worse, the reeds as well as the body of the instrument continue to change even while the instrumentalist is trying to adjust his techniques for playing on it.

Most of the changes in voice are completed within a 6-month period. However, for a variety of reasons, including some that may be psychological, the changes or the adjustments to the changes may go on for a year or more.

What are the parents' responsibilities for the boy or girl whose voice is "not right" for 6 months or more into the period of obvious physiological adolescence? Usually, sympathetic understanding is enough on the positive side. Teasing, even when allegedly good humored and "for fun," is definitely to be avoided. If the adolescent's voice seems to be settling down, with fewer breaks and fewer uncontrollable changes in pitch and quality, then all you need is patience. What should be happening is happening, and all is going well.

Suppose, however, that either the boy or girl is trying to sound like a preadolescent child. The voice tends to be a falsetto, high in pitch, but without the quality of the child's voice. This may suggest that the physically adolescent boy or girl may still want or need to be a preadolescent child. We strongly recommend, however, that this possible conclusion not be made by the parents or any other relative. It should be made only by a *physician who understands young adolescents and their growing-up problems.* Parents should seek advice of such a physician. If the physician recommends counseling or

---

[5]The analogy to string instruments may be misleading. The voice mechanism is really more like a wind instrument. The vocal folds (cords) or " voice lips" are similar to the reeds of wind instruments. The cavities of the windpipe (larynx), throat, mouth, and nasal cavities reinforce the tones, much as the body of the wind instrument reinforces the tones of the vibrating reeds. Air (breath), under the control of the musician or speaker, sets the reeds or vocal folds into vibration and creates the identifying sound of the instrument or voice.

psychotherapy, follow this advice. But do assure your adolescent that he or she is not abnormal or neurotic or in any way sick, but rather needs help to get over the voice problem.

If the physician sees no indication of any growing-up problem, the adolescent may be helped by a voice therapist who *specializes in the speaking voice.* Let me emphasize that you should get medical clearance from the boy's or girl's physician, or from a laryngologist, before any voice training is undertaken.

In general, even when there are no serious problems, parents need to keep in mind the close relationship between voice and emotions in their adolescents. Voice reflects slight changes in stress, and adolescence is a period of stress. The voice that reflects this state of feeling is not abnormal. If any treatment is indicated at all, it should be in the direction of reducing stress. If reducing stress is not possible, an attitude of understanding will help. You don't need to verbalize this understanding unless the adolescent asks for it. A sensitive adolescent will be aware of your attitude and be grateful for it.

When the male adolescent has learned to control his muscles and has learned to adapt to the changes in the vocal mechanism, he will be able to control the pitch and quality of his voice. This may take from 6 to 18 months. Patience is needed, both by the parent for the male adolescent and by the adolescent for himself. As noted, voice changes for girls are less cataclysmic.

The vocal mechanism is essentially a wind instrument. As children, we learn to play the tiny instruments fairly effectively if we have proper models. As adolescents, we may again have to learn how to play our instrument. Once more, as in early childhood, a poor model may make it difficult for us to adjust to the instrument or to attain an effective voice. But most of us, somehow, become fairly proficient vocal instrumentalists, at least for speaking, and all goes well. A fortunate few become virtuosos and learn to produce voices that are not only effective but also beautiful.

In the absence of physical or psychological problems, almost all children are capable of developing a moderately effective voices. "Moderately effective" means that the voice should be appropriate to the age, gender, and physical features of the child, the adolescent, and ultimately the adult. An acceptable voice should

- be pleasant, or at least not unpleasant, to hear;
- reflect changes in feeling and thinking through pitch range, loudness, and quality; and

- be produced without discomfort and fatigue (although fatigue and discomfort may set in with prolonged speaking).

If your child's voice meets these standards, it is a normal voice. How does your own voice measure up? A special note for adolescents: To have an effective voice, you must use your *own* voice and not that of a person you may admire. Your voice mechanism has its own unique physical properties. Make the most of them!

The selected readings for this chapter, listed in Appendix 11A, are those of authorities on children's voices. A few are technical, but none are too difficult for the layperson to understand.

Appendix 11A
Selected List of Readings
on Children's Voices

Boone, D. R., & McFarlane, S. C. (1984). *The voice and voice therapy* (5th ed.). Englewood Cliffs, NJ: Prentice-Hall. (This is a technical but clearly written textbook on the normal voice and psychological and physical causes of disorders of voice, including those of children. Excellent illustrations.)

DeVilliers, P. A., & DeVilliers, J. G. (1979). *Early language.* Cambridge, MA: Harvard University Press. (The authors explain how even at the one-word stage, children use differences in intonation to signal the different meanings of the utterance. A delightful book to read and study.)

Eisenson, J., & Ogilivie, M. (1983). *Communication disorders in children* (5th ed.). New York: Macmillan. (This is an introductory textbook intended for students who are planning to become speech–language clinicians. Because the book employs a minimum of technical language, it is appropriate for lay readers and for clinicians who may be consulted on problems of speech and voice. The authors emphasize the role that the classroom teacher and the parent play in the understanding of problems in communication, including those that are caused by voice disorders.)

Fernald, A. (1982, February 8). *Parent's melodies as key to conveying the lyrics of language.* Paper presented at a meeting of the American Association for the Advancement of Science, Chicago. (Dr. Fernald, a psychologist, explains how parents use voice melodies, long pauses, and word stretches to help get the attention of babies—to communicate and teach them language.)

Greene, M. (1980). *The voice and its disorders.* Philadelphia: Lippincott. (Though on the technical side, the author presents clear and brief explanations of the most frequent voice disorders in children and adults.)

Harris, M. (1987). The relationship of maternal speech to children's first words. In D. J. Messer & G. F. Turner (Eds.), *Critical influences on child language acquisition and development.* New York: St. Martin's Press. (In her contribution to this book, Harris discusses the relationship of maternal speech to children's first words.)

Wilson, D. K. (1987). *Voice problems of children.* Baltimore: Williams & Wilkins. (This is a somewhat technical explanation of the voice problems of children, but it is balanced by easy-to-understand suggestions for approaches to therapy and treatment.)

Wood, B. S. (1981). *Children and communication.* Englewood Cliffs, NJ: Prentice-Hall. (In the chapter "The Child's Voice Communicates," the author explains that "the voice is a powerful channel for communicating ideas, feelings, and attitudes, both obvious and subtle" (p. 198). She also notes that *prosody,* the music of our speech, is "the earliest dimension of language to be employed and understood by infants" (p. 199). Wood believes that "the babbled utterances contain the prosodic features of the full-fledged sentences that adults use" (p. 199).

Chapter 12

Is My Child
Delayed in Speech?

Thus far most of our discussions have focused on normal speech and language development. The chapters on cluttering and stuttering were the exceptions. Some of our discussions may not have been explicit or direct. In this chapter we will be both explicit and direct in answering the question "Is my child delayed in speech?"

Except for children who are deaf, who use a sign language system, speech is a word-of-mouth language product. Words consist of selected sounds and combinations of sounds that are used in a particular language system such as English, French, Spanish, German, or Chinese. The form, or structure, of the words, as well as the selection and combination of sounds that indicate meanings, varies with each language.

The "rules" that determine how we arrange words in a sentence are known as "grammar" or "syntax." Each language has its own rules. We may refer to the selection of words and grammar as a "language code." A child who is delayed in speaking may be slow in understanding the code. Or, he or she may understand the code—sometimes revealing this understanding by his or her appropriate behavior—but he or she may nonetheless be significantly delayed in speaking. However, keep in mind that it is both usual and normal for a child to indicate comprehension weeks to months before saying first readily comprehensible words (even though the words may include "baby" sounds). Failure to understand speech, provided that the content is not lengthy or complex (review our discussion of "motherese"), carries much more serious implications of delay than does tardiness in speech production. At the risk of being blunt, we will now answer the question of the title of this chapter.

When Is Speech Delayed?

Despite the newborn infant's attention and bonding with human vocalizers, we do not expect newborn infants to understand what we say to or at them. This is so even though the vast majority of children are born with the capacity, or instinct, for language, and, of course, the potential to become listeners and speakers in their own right. Thus, beyond their urgent biological needs, which have their own signals in the various types of crying, caring adults anticipate needs and respond to them. But there does come a time when we expect babies to understand some of what we say to them, to begin to decode our spoken language system. There also comes a time when we expect them to use their mouths for something beyond eating, gurgling, crying, and laughing. When should this time be?

If infants were statistics, we could answer this question with considerable assurance. In Chapter 2 we noted that some children (more likely girls than boys) say their first words before the end of the first year. A small percentage may even use words to name a few objects or persons as early as 7 or 8 months. But most children don't say intelligible words until they are between 12 and 15 months of age. A few don't begin to talk until they are almost 24 months old. And a very small percentage may not say their first words until they are 30 months of age.

Who, if any, of the children in these age groups shall we consider delayed? Certainly not the children who understand speech and say their first words by 15 months. Is 2 years delayed? Perhaps, because purely on the basis of statistics, most children—that is, more than 50%—say their first words by 18 months. But a human infant should not be treated as a statistic unless we play the number game intelligently. There are late talkers just as there are late walkers, late jumpers, late tricycle riders, and late block builders. Fortunately, in adjusting to the numbers game we can take comfort from the fact that many "latenesses" run in families.

A child may start to speak later than all other children of the same age and gender. Nevertheless, if that child comes from a family in which daddy, grandaddy, and Uncle Joe had nothing to say (or at any rate said nothing) until 24 months or even as late as 30 months, there is no great cause for concern. If, however, the child does not understand sentences, especially simple sentences made up of words that name things and actions that are part of everyday life, we would be concerned regardless of the family picture. Even a slow-to-speak child should understand, "Open your mouth," or "Here's your dolly," and respond appropriately.

Comprehension does not necessarily imply that the child responds affirmatively. A negative response such as a tightening of the jaws to the request of "open your mouth" may indicate understanding, but, for whatever reason or nonreason the child entertains at the moment, it may be an expression of negative feeling about the "command." So might a poke at the dolly's eyes express comprehension and feeling. Just why even the best of children decide on occasion to be noncompliant is another matter, which we will not undertake to explain here.

The 18- to 24-Month Period

There is something of magic in this critical 18- to 24-month language-development period. A child may enter this stage with his or her first intelligible words, or a vocabulary of from 5 to 10 words. At the end of this 6-month period, the child may have anywhere from 50 to several hundred words. Moreover, when the child has a vocabulary of 50 or more speaking words, he or she usually begins to combine words into phrase-sentences. These may begin with "big boy," "baby cookie," or "that dog." As this vocabulary grows, and the child increases the number of words in these phrase-sentences, we may hear "girl fall down," "look in it," and "me jump up." At the outset of this critical age period, the child refers to himself or herself either by the name used by others or as "me." At the end of the period, the child understands "I" and the difference between you, me, and I. Usually the child uses the highly personal pronoun "I" as appropriately as adults do.

With these references to vocabulary size and word phrases, we have another way of looking at and measuring language delay. We noted that most children combine words into phrase-sentences when they have a basic vocabulary of about 50 words. Children who are not using two-word combinations by the time that their base vocabulary has reached 100 words may certainly be considered as delayed.

Note that we are no longer referring to the age of the child but to the size and growth of vocabulary. This approach to viewing language development and language delay permits us to distinguish between the late-to-start child who catches up and those who do not. To restate the difference, the physically and mentally normal child who is a late starter catches up with the early starters. Children who are delayed do not and continue to be slow in their language development. The gaps tend to close between 36 to 42 months. However, very early starters—those below 12 months of age, and especially those of superior intelligence—are likely to have good home stimulation and so stay out front. The greatest differences will be in the size of vocabulary and their capacity to understand and deal with abstract concepts.

The 24- to 36-Month Period

The 18- to 24-month period is usually considered crucial for language development. During this period, the child goes from words to phrase-sentences. The next period, from 24 to 36 months, usually brings great acceleration and achievement in language. The child has figured out the code. Speaking vocabulary may increase from 100 words to 1,000 words. By 36 months, many of the sentences the child uses are as grammatical as those of the adults who talk to the child. Moreover, almost everything the child says is *intelligible,* not only to those with whom the child lives but also to strangers.

We now have another way to tell when speech is delayed. This concerns *intelligibility,* which we first considered in Chapter 7. Now we need to differentiate *distinctly* from *intelligibly.* A child may say a certain sound without the proper articulation, or may slur one syllable of a word, yet the sentence as a whole may be intelligible. I am not by any means recommending indistinct speaking. But I do wish to point out that intelligibility alone can be a measure of speech development.

Of course, good articulation and intelligibility are related. Speech that has sloppy articulation is both indistinct *and* unintelligible. But a child of 3 years may be highly intelligible, even if he or she does not have all the sounds and sound blends of the language under control. When a child has a vocabulary of 1,000 words or more—this may be at about 3 years of age—we should expect intelligibility. This does not mean complete control over the individual sounds or sound blends. The child may also understand hundreds of words spoken to him or her, but these may not be ready for use. Comprehension exceeds production at all ages.

Most normal children have control of vowel sounds early in their speech development and usually by the age of 4 years. This is in contrast with the control of the consonants. This is so because the vowel sounds are all produced with voice and are louder in context than are consonants. Vowels are also more distinguishable one from another than are many of the consonants. Although each child has his or her own schedule for speech sound control, there are some general parameters (see Table 12.1). We will consider control as established if the child produces the appropriate sound in his or her speech more than 50% of the time.

Speech sound control sometimes may lapse and revert to an earlier stage of pronunciation. It may be that, for reasons not always evident to the parents, the child is expressing a desire for "the good old days" before age 2 or 3 years. We may see this acted out when a child, more likely a girl than a boy, attributes baby talk to a favorite doll or a teddy bear during play. The arrival of a new member of the family may trigger off baby talk. These and other possibilities should be discussed with the child's pediatrician before the parents involve the child in speech sound correction.

Frequent Articulation "Errors"

Frequent articulation "errors" for children from age 2 to 7 years are as follows:

- Sounds that are close together in manner of production may be interchanged. For example, *p* and *b, t,* and *k* may give us *pandy* or *tandy* for *candy; doggy* may become *doddy* or *bobby.*

- A sound, especially one that is newly "controlled," may be used more than once in a word, as in the examples above. Thus a dolly (newly controlled *l*) may become *lolly;* a *kitty* may become *kicky* or *titty.* These are usually short-term productions.

- As a general rule, sounds controlled early may be substituted for later controlled sounds. Table 12.1 may serve as a guide for these substitutions.

- A child's perception of sounds in context may be closer to what is actually produced by adults than we assume. In context, *an apple* is

Table 12.1
Usual Age (in Years) for Control
of the Consonants of English

Age Range	Sounds
2–3	*p, m, n, h, w, b, k, t, d, g, ng* (as in *wing*)
3–4	*f, y, l, s*
4–5	*r, ch, sh, z, j* (as in *jump*), *v*
5–6	*th* as in *thin, th* as in *that*
6–7	*zh* as in *measure,* and all of the above

Note. Adapted from "When Are Speech Sounds Learned?" by E. K. Sander (1972), *Journal of Speech and Hearing Disorders, 37,* p. 62.

actually pronounced as *a napple* and *an orange* as *a norange.* The trusting child therefore calls these fruits *napple* and *norange.*

- The sequence of syllables in multisyllable words may be produced with the syllables out of order. Thus, the favorite *spaghetti* may become *gasphetti* and an *elephant* an *efalent.* Unless these become family words, the correct syllable sequence is under control in a few months. But *aks* for *ask* may be considerably more resistant.

Table 12.1 is intended as a guide to the usual ages for the control of the consonants of American English. It should not be viewed as a rigid table of expectancies. Girls may be ahead of these age expectancies. Early starters are likely to be advanced in speech sound control. In any event, a plus-or-minus 6 to 9 months would be sufficiently approximate for most children with the exception of those who have a significant hearing loss in the speech sound range.

Bilingualism

In general, in regard to language development, is there an advantage or disadvantage for a child to be brought up in a home where more than one language is spoken? The answer is a conditional "yes" and may also be a conditional "no." The primary conditional reservation is, "How proficient are the speakers in each of the languages?" If the parents, or other key members of the family, are truly bilingual—can speak and think comfortably and well in each of the languages—the child may acquire comparable proficiency. As a point of interest, a child who is brought up in such a home is likely to be able to switch from one language to another until about age 2 years, without being aware of the switching. The child is likely to respond in the language addressed to him or her. There is no recorded evidence of any disadvantage to such language exposure.

The conditional "no" is for homes in which there is uneven proficiency between the two languages. The child is at a disadvantage if the key members of the family are proficient in their first (native) language but not comparably proficient in the second. If, however, the family includes a member who is proficient in the second language, interchange with this speaker may provide some of the advantages of bilingualism.[1]

Another approach to teaching a second language before the child enters school is to engage a person who is proficient in the language as a caregiver for the child. This obviously implies a degree of economic affluence not available to all homes. Traditionally, this was a practice of European families for teaching a child a selected second language. A nurse or nanny was the caregiver and also the teacher of the selected language by appropriate talking while doing whatever was necessary for the child.

Another approach used in some private schools in the United States and Canada is to devote given parts of the day for teaching a subject consistently in the desired second language. In Canada, it is French; in the United States it is usually Spanish. Such an arrangement permits the pupils to have a "set" and expectation during the school day. One truly bilingual family in my academic community speaks English at one mealtime and French during dinner. The child is at school for lunch and there speaks English.

If the child shows significant delay in understanding and speaking, then I suggest that only one language be spoken in the home. Bilingual exposure for late starters may cause confusion and overall delay. If the child is a member of a family with siblings or close relatives who are or were slow-to-start speakers, one language at a time is enough. (I review the subject and issues of second language learning in Chapters 7 and 9 of Eisenson and Ogilvie, 1983, *Communication Disorders in Children.*)

---

[1] I am intentionally avoiding the ongoing debates about bilingual teaching in the schools of the United States. This is not a concern of the issues related to language delay in this book.

Why Doesn't My Child Listen?
Hearing and Listening

At the outset, we must distinguish between possible problems in listening and hearing and willfully not listening. Let us assume that there is no reason to suspect that a child has a hearing loss—that the child can hear sounds, including those of speech, but does not choose to "tune in" to you to hear (listen) to you. He or she may be involved in a game or looking at or possibly reading a book, or watching a favorite program on television. The child may hear your voice, but is too occupied to listen. Listening is a responsible act that requires figuring out your message (decoding) and doing something about it. Not seeming to hear is for the moment a release from responsibility. This is normal behavior and not limited to children. When the child is ready—soon, we hope—he or she is yours again for both hearing and listening.

Now let us take 2-year-old Joel, who has no apparent difficulty in hearing his dog bark, his cat meow, and the canary sing in its cage. He indicates this ability by turning in the direction of each of these sound makers and may play verbally with his pets. But he does not answer when you ask, "Do you want to feed the canary?" unless he can see you with the canary food in hand. He may turn to you for a moment and then turn away unless there is a visible cue for him to "read" the situation. Even if we allow for occasional negative behavior, Joel's underlying problem is one of listening. The child seems to be unable to make sense out of a flow of spoken language—technically, to decode the flow of language when it is produced at a normal rate of production.

A technical term for this listening problem is *central auditory disorder.* The term *central* implies that there is either a delay in the maturation of the areas of the brain that "specialize" in the comprehension of spoken language or possibly of brain damage to those language areas (see Figure 10.1).[2] By "early damage," I mean incurred before the age when children normally begin to understand and soon after to say their first words. The age of these abilities varies from 8 to 18 months and should be approximated by comparison with siblings or with closely related children. Another term for central auditory disorder is *developmental childhood dysphasia* (Eisenson & Ogilvie, 1983).

---

[2]This discussion is essentially an expansion of the one on attention-deficit disorders in Chapter 10. However, children with central auditory disorder are not necessarily hyperactive.

In some instances, children with central auditory disorder (CAD) give the impression of being deaf, at least to spoken language—and will make no attempt to listen. In effect, they may hear but cannot attend because of their decoding problem. If the child is punished by frustrated and puzzled parents who do not understand how a child can respond to nonhuman sounds and not to persons who speak to them, the child may turn away from all sound makers and withdraw into him- or herself. Professional treatment for such children is fortunately both available and most often successful. Treatment should include parent counseling.

Although the following is not intended as a substitute for professional help, these basic suggestions should be helpful to parents. Pretend that your child is about 18 months of age. Address the child in simple sentences. In fact, begin with single words that refer to objects, parts of the body, toys, and pets. While facing a mirror, point to and identify (say) "nose" (yours and his or hers). Repeat this several times, at first asking only that he or she points to the nose. When you are satisfied that the youngster understands, try the single-word statement with one or two pictures of children that have an easily identifiable nose. Then say "nose" and wait for the child to point. Again, repeat the performance with just the word, and wait for the child to point. (You will, of course, say or do something rewarding for each correct effort. This is the old M & M approach, which does not necessarily require candy.)

At this stage, we are primarily concerned with establishing listening and word comprehension. If the child says the word—and it need not be sound perfect; baby pronunciation will do—you will, of course, indicate your pleasure. Now you are ready to move on to two-word statements that make use of the word or words the child understands. If it is still a matter of nose, we have "mommy nose," "daddy nose," "Bobby [child's name] nose," and so on. You must be patient and appreciate that repetition is important. But do not produce your repetitions in rapid sequence; a short pause and *slow but not distorted pronunciation* is desired. Exaggerate your speech melody (intonation) and speak more slowly than you would to an older child, your spouse, or a friend. Avoid a tendency to shout. Remember, your child is not deaf but has a listening problem!

I am intentionally not going beyond these minimal suggestions because of my strong belief that the child with central auditory disorder or developmental dysphasia should be seen by a professional clinician. Your own role as a parent should be what your clinician advises. Your child's pediatrician or family physician should be able to direct you to a certified clinician. (Chapter 13 of this book focuses on where to go for help.)

Acquired Dysphasia

Acquired dysphasia is an impairment in the ability to understand or to speak after these language abilities have been established. This impairment may be the result of injury or disease to the parts of the cortex (top layer of the brain) that are devoted to language. For almost all right-handed children, this would be the left half of the cortex. For a small minority of children who are left-handed, the damage may be in the right half of the cortex.

Depending on the level of language proficiency reached by the child at the age of the brain damage, the child will lose that level of ability and may for a short time seem to be mute, or to resort to single words or frustrated gestures. Fortunately, young brains are elastic, so that alternate parts of the brain or the other half (hemisphere) may take over the role of the normally dominant one for language. In general, as the child recovers physically from the "insult" to the brain, he or she also makes rapid recovery from the language impairments. The outlook is favorable for virtually complete language recovery. In states of excitement, fatigue, or an unrelated illness, some of the language problems may recur. Residual problems, such as not finding the right word, incorrect grammatical constructions, and pronunciation and articulation difficulties may be present for a time, in some instances for several months, after the onset of the damage and language disruption. Generally, however, the recovery outlook is favorable and for most children, virtually complete.

Other residual problems may become evident in school learning. A child who has learned to read may have difficulties in reading at expected grade level. Spelling errors may occur more frequently than before the language disruption. Mathematics beyond simple arithmetic may be a problem. For most postdysphasic children, these problems are overcome, and the child is likely to come close to early expectations. This is especially so if the dysphasia occurs before age 9 or 10 years. It is also so for a majority of children up to the age of adolescence.

In the next chapter, we present information on where to go for professional help.

Appendix 12A
Selected List of Readings on Language Delay

Selecting readings for the following list was difficult not because there are so few sources, but because there are so many. The other problem is that most of the publications are rather technical and do not make for easy reading. My decisions are based on the references I knew best and that are least likely to be beyond the needs of the readers of this book.

Bates, E., Bretherton, I., & Snyder, L. (1988). *From first words to grammar.* New York: Cambridge University Press. (The underlying theme of this book is that children do not learn language the same way. Chapter 16 addresses the differences in learning two languages simultaneously.)

Davis, J., & Hardick, E. J. (1981). *Rehabilitation audiology for children and adults.* New York: Wiley. (This book deals with language learning of children with hearing loss. Chapter 5 deals with intervention programs. The book is well illustrated and relatively easy to read.)

deVilliers, P. A., & deVilliers, J. G. (1979). *Early language.* Cambridge, MA: Harvard University Press. (This decidedly easy-to-read book deals for the most part with the early language development of two children, the authors' own. Chapter 8 is concerned with restraints in language learning. Dysphasia is briefly mentioned.)

Eisenson, J. (1984). *Aphasia and related disorders in children.* New York: Harper & Row. (This is devoted to the diagnosis and treatment of children with language problems resulting from brain damage. The book includes a large section on therapeutic approaches.)

Eisenson, J. (1984). *Reading for meaning: An illustrated language acquisition program.* Tulsa, OK: Modern Education Corp.

Eisenson, J. (1997). *ILAP: An illustrated language acquisition program.* Manuscript in preparation.

Eisenson, J., & Ogilvie, M. (1983). *Communication disorders in children* (5th ed.). New York: Macmillan. (This is an introductory book on communication disorders that includes several chapters on normal and delayed language development, impaired hearing, and brain differences and acquired aphasia. Though intended for the classroom teacher, much of the content is directed toward the parent and the contributions of the home to improving the communication problems of children.)

Katz, J., Stetker, N., & Henderson, D. (Eds.). (1992). *Central auditory processing.* St. Louis, MO: C. V. Mosby. (The editors express the hope that their book will provide readers with useful ideas to consider in their work with children who have central auditory processing impairment. They also provide useful techniques and approaches for evaluating and remediating CAPD.)

Keath, R. W. (Ed.). (1981). *Central auditory and language disorders in children.* Houston, TX: College Hill Press. (Several chapters in this multiauthored book by authorities in the field of language disorders deal with the varied aspects of language processing disorders.)

U.S. General Service Administration. (1996). *Consumer information catalogue.* Pueblo, CO: Consumer Information Center. (This agency offers free booklets and other materials at very low prices on many subjects, including learning disabilities and language and reading skills. Address: Consumer Information Center, Pueblo, CO 81002.)

Van Riper, C., & Emerick, L. (1984). *Speech correction* (7th ed.). Englewood Cliffs, NJ: Prentice-Hall. (An introductory textbook that is well within the comprehension abilities of most lay persons. Developmental language problems, hearing problems, and aphasia [dysphasia] are discussed in separate chapters.)

Chapter 13

When and Where
To Go for Help

It is a rare child whose early words are pronounced as he or she will pronounce words 2 years after starting out in the acquisition of spoken language. Early language up to at least age 3 is characterized by baby talk. Unless this persists despite increases in spoken vocabulary and grammatical productions, there is neither need nor cause for concern. In fact, early intervention may create self-consciousness about speaking, with possible negative effects. Even early dysfluencies in speaking are usually passing expressions of reaching for new words or new "grammatical" ways of making statements and/or asking questions. The exceptions may be children who come from a family of identified stutterers. Such children may be helped by efforts to organize units of language that seem to be associated with dysfluency in production. (See discussion on early stuttering in Chapter 9.)

In general, we expect, or at least hope, that professional speech–language clinicians share this view. If so, when consulted by an anxious parent, the advice would be that intervention is not heeded nor desirable, and to let normal development take its course.

Then, when is early intervention necessary? We have already touched on stuttering. Problems that have a physical basis may justify intervention. Such problems include vocal nodules, hearing loss, neurological impairments, and clefts of the mouth and palate. Children with oral clefts are the primary concern of the oral surgeon, who should determine when speech intervention is to be initiated.

Children with basic medical or physical conditions should be "cleared" by their pediatrician or family physician or medical specialist to determine readiness for speech or language intervention.

Now, where to go for help? In the United States, the majority of speech–language clinicians (speech pathologists)—professionally educated and trained persons—are likely to be members of the American Speech-Language-Hearing Association (ASHA). In Canada, clinicians may be members of parallel associations as well as ASHA. In both the United States and Canada, there are also many regional and local organizations.

The national organizations have certification procedures and award certificates of clinical competence to applicants who meet certification requirements. These requirements include appropriate education, supervised clinical experience, and an examination. To be sure, on an individual basis certification does not guarantee competence, but it is a major step in that direction.

In the United States, many states have licensing requirements that are much like those for ASHA certification. A physician, psychologist, or other family consultant who wishes to make a referral to a speech–language clinician or hearing specialist (audiologist) may inquire of any state or regional organization or directly of ASHA for names of certified personnel.

Outside of the United States and Canada, many countries have professional associations or colleges that parallel ASHA in certification responsibilities and also provide education and training. For example, Great Britain and Australia have colleges of speech therapy with courses that lead to certification. In several European countries, medical specialists called "phoniatrists" and nonmedically educated clinicians called "logopedists" provide speech and language therapy.

In the United States, professional services are available in public as well as many private universities and colleges that have educational programs for clinicians as well as supervised training clinics. Usual names for such departments are "Speech Pathology and Audiology," "Speech and Hearing Disorders," and "Communication Disorders." These departments may also have listings of qualified (certified) clinicians. In some instances, there are therapy units within a department of otolaryngology (ear, throat). Some universities have separate schools for academic training of speech clinicians and audiologists that include clinical services.

Most public schools provide therapy from the primary to the secondary grades. Medical centers, both public and private, may provide therapeutic services.

I shall restate my position in regard to medical clearance—a point that I cannot overemphasize. Children, and adults for that matter, who have voice problems *should be cleared by a physician before treatment for the symptoms are undertaken.* This clearance also holds for any physical problem and for readiness for symptom treatment. Periodic consultation with the physician is strongly recommended.

Epilogue

As you are reading these words, you are taking part in one of the wonders of the natural world. For you and I belong to a species with a remarkable ability: we can shape events in each other's brains with exquisite precision. . . . Simply by making noises with our mouths, we can reliably cause precise new combinations of ideas to arise in each other's minds. The ability comes so naturally that we are apt to forget what a miracle it is.

STEVEN PINKER, *THE LANGUAGE INSTINCT*

We do not know how spoken language originated, nor do we know whether in the history of humanity there was once a single language or whether there were several languages that originated and developed in different parts of the world at the same time or over long periods of years. Nor do we know just how languages took their form, how they became symbol systems that included rules for speaking and listening, rules that could be encoded and decoded. But we do know that somehow almost all children discover language for themselves. We may call this recurring miracle the *language instinct.* In expressing this instinct, children create their own language. In this creation, the language each child speaks is remarkably like the language of their elders in most instances, but remarkably unlike in some instances, and more like that of peers or that of older siblings. Somehow, the spoken language also manages to express the child's own individuality as a human being.

Very early in their careers as speakers, children learn how much broader potential language is than serving as a device for extending their limited physical reach, for getting things out of sight but not out of mind. Language is for thinking, for telling important truths, and sometimes for deceiving persons who, at least for the moment, are important to deceive.

Language is also for making secrets through inventing words that you share with someone very, very special. And language is for playing, for making sounds that go beyond the mere need to make sense.

In time, we learn the importance of the trivial, of what words we need to use—and how to use them—for social contact. We also learn something children appreciate, the "rules" for turn taking. A mouthful of unspoken words is hard to digest.

Soon, perhaps never too soon, children learn what Washington Irving observed in *Rip Van Winkle:* "A sharp tongue is the only edged tool that grows keener with constant use." If fortunate, the child, when grown and mature as an adult, can rejoice with William Blake:

> When the voices of children are heard on the green
> And laughter is heard on the hill
> My heart is at rest within my breast
> And everything else is still.

References

American Psychiatric Association. (1980). *Diagnostic and statistical manual of mental disorders* (3rd ed.). Washington, DC: Author.

American Psychiatric Association. (1994). *Diagnostic and statistical manual of mental disorders* (4th ed.). Washington, DC: Author.

Baron, N. (1992). *Growing up with language.* Reading, MA: Addison Wesley.

Bellugi, U. (1970, December). Learning the language. *Psychology Today, 4.*

Bowlby, J. (1958). The nature of the child's tie to the mother. *International Journal of Psychoanalysis, 39,* 350–373.

Bruner, J. (1975). The ontogenesis of speech acts. *Journal of Child Language, 2,* 1–19.

Bruner, J. (1983). *Child's talk.* New York, W. W. Norton.

Cheng, L.-R. L. (1991). *Assessing Asian language performance.* Oceanside, CA: Academic Communication Associates.

Clark, R. (1971). *Einstein: Life and times.* New York: World Publishing Co.

Davis, H., & Silverman, S. R. (1978). *Hearing and deafness.* New York: Holt, Rinehart & Winston.

Davis, J. M., & Hardick, E. D. (1981). *Rehabilitation audiology in children and adults.* New York: Wiley.

DeCasper, A. J., & Fifer, W. P. (1980). Of human bondage. Newborns prefer their mothers' voices. *Science, 208,* 1174–1176.

DeVilliers, P. A., & DeVilliers, J. G. (1979). *Early language.* Cambridge, MA: Harvard University Press.

Education for All Handicapped Children Act of 1975, 20 U.S.C. § 1400 *et seq.*

Eisenson, J. (1984). *Aphasia and related disorders in children* (2nd ed.). New York: Harper & Row.

Eisenson, J. (1989). *Language and speech disorders in children.* New York: Pergamon.

Eisenson, J. (1997). *ILAP: An illustrated language acquisition program.* Manuscript in preparation.

Eisenson, J., & Ogilvie, M. (1983). *Communicative disorders in children* (5th ed.). New York: Macmillan.

Eisenson, J., & Ogilvie, M. (1988). *Communicative disorders in children* (6th ed.). New York: Macmillan.

Fernald, A. C. (1989). Intonation and communicative intent in mothers' speech to infants: Is the melody the message? *Child Development, 6,* 1497–1510.

Furth, H. G. (1973). *Deafness and learning.* Belmont, CA: Wadsworth.

Halliday, M. A. K. (1975). *Learning how to mean.* London: Edward Arnold.

Harris, M. (1987). The relationship of maternal speech to children's first words. In D. J. Messer & G. F. Turner (Eds.), *Critical influences on child language acquisition and development.* New York: St Martin's.

Ingram, D., & Eisenson, J. (1972). *Aphasia in children.* New York: Harper.

Lewis, M. M. (1951). *Infant speech.* New York: Humanities Press.

Lieberman, P. (1966). *Intonation, perception, and language.* Cambridge, MA: MIT Press.

Kinsbourne, M., & Caplan, P. (1979). *Children's learning and attention deficits.* Boston: Little, Brown.

Klaus, M. H., & Klaus, P. H. (1985). *The amazing newborn.* Reading, MA: Addison Wesley.

Martin, F. N. (1986). *Introduction to audiology* (3d ed.). Englewood Cliffs, NJ: Prentice-Hall.

Ornstein, R., & Thompson, R. (1984). *The amazing brain.* Boston: Houghton Mifflin.

Pinker, S. (1994). *The language instinct.* New York: Morrow.

Renfrew, C., & Murphy, K. (1964). *The child who does not talk.* London: Heinemann.

Ross, D. A. (1977). *Auditory perception of speech.* Englewood Cliffs, NJ: Prentice-Hall.

Sander, E. K. (1972). When are speech sounds learned? *Journal of Speech and Hearing Disorders, 37,* 54–63.

Stocker, B., & Goldfarb, R. (1995). *The Stocker probe technique* (3rd ed.). Vera Beach, FL: Speed Bin.

Van Riper, C. (1950). *Teaching your child to talk.* New York: Harper & Row.

Wasz-Hockert, J., Lind, V., Vuorenkoski, V., Partenen, T., & Valanne, E. (1968). *The infant cry.* New York: Lippincott.

Weissbluth, M. (1984). *Crybabies.* New York: Arbor House.

Index

NOTES

NOTES

NOTES

NOTES